There's a Rooster in My Bathroom!

A Quest for Meaning in the Bathroom, the Boardroom and Beyond

Trish Ostroski

Dedication to the Readers

Life Lessons and the Meaning of Life
For *Liviu* and Everyone Else

Stories from the Peace Corps, Earthquakes, Career, Arts,
Hollywood and More

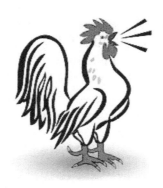

They are Crowing Praises for --

There's a Rooster in My Bathroom!

A Quest for Meaning in the Bathroom,

the Boardroom and Beyond

"A beautiful, daily book-on-the-nightstand read!

Trish "rings the bell" (as she did in the Peace Corps) with insights and observations from a life lived from Moldova to Hollywood and beyond, and she shares her wonderful ride!"

Joan van Ark
Actress

"As a speaker/trainer, I encourage my clients to "Speak from the Heart." Share their stories. The stories which offer insight and life lessons for their audiences. That is exactly what you get with Trish Ostroski's *There's A Rooster in My Bathroom*.

Throughout this thought-provoking book, Trish provides a variety of stories that will be valued by many and covering various facets of life. I especially liked the chapter "Right

Time to Lose Your Job" because she illustrates what might be considered by many as a setback but how she writes…Can be a fresh journey to a new adventure. What I like best about this chapter as well as for the rest of the book, Trish offers examples of what you can do to better your life. You are going to enjoy reading AND applying the lessons in this whimsical, easy to read book. Enjoy!"

Maurice DiMino
International Award-Winning Speaker
MauriceDiMino.com

"Trish's career focused on service above self, which allowed her to experiences places and people most of us only dream of. Her stories will resonate with anyone who loves travel and life lessons learned on the journey."

Kyle Kutuchief
Program Director in Akron
for Knight Foundation

Reading Trish Ostroski's *There's a Rooster in my Bathroom!*, reads as I imagine most tales of a life well- lived should, like scenes from a movie. Each one captures a different aspect of the life lived by Trish, allowing the reader to page through each section as it captures their interest. I am a musician, so I really enjoyed the section where she got to attend a seminar by Janis Ian, who guided Trish and others through the meaning of her song, "At Seventeen," line by line. What a night that must have been! I highly recommend *There's a Rooster in my Bathroom* for anyone who loves a good story! You won't regret it!

Mark Brown
Musician, Community Theater actor and director

"Trish Ostroski's *There's a Rooster in my Bathroom*! is a wonderful group of stories about her Peace Corps experiences that offers life lessons for any reader. It's proof again that the most compelling way to learn about other people and places is through skilled story telling.

Her recollections of a boy named Liviu particularly touched me and illuminated the perspective a child can bring to facing life's challenges. I know from my 40 years of serving as CEO of Akron Children's Hospital how true this is. Trish's collection of stories is thoughtful, real and written in an easy to read style. Enjoy!

William H. Considine
CEO Emeritus
Akron Children's Hospital

There's A Rooster in My Bathroom! is a delightful and refreshing read! Trish's true stories are both captivating and insightful. I couldn't stop reading of her tales, trials and tribulations. I appreciated the synchronicity and spiritual awareness in the lessons shared throughout the book. As Trish reminds us, sharing our stories is important — and adds to our humanity. I'm inspired!"

Sheryl Roush
CEO Sparkle Presentations, Inc
SherylRoush.com

There's a Rooster in My Bathroom!

A Quest for Meaning in the Bathroom, the Boardroom and Beyond

Trish Ostroski

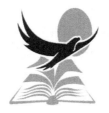

Paperback ISBN: 978-1-64184-103-0

eBook ISBN: 978-1-64184-104-7

The Piper Has Called

As we go to press on this book, my brother Mark Ostroski climbed the *stairway to heaven* on June 1, 2019. MarkO was the strong middle branch of our family as the sixth child in a family of eleven siblings. He had an infectious, trademark laugh and hailed his four basic food groups as being cookies, cake, ice cream, and soda pop. The music he loved was food for his spirit. His laughter and jokes were food for our souls. Congratulations, MarkO. Job well done. You have climbed that *stairway to heaven* and enjoy your new journey.

This book includes the complete lyrics to

At Seventeen

composed by Janis Ian

This book contains the play

See You Sooner

By Trish Ostroski

Introduction

Life Lessons

I served in the United States Peace Corps from 2013-2015 in Moldova in Eastern Europe. Moldova is Europe's poorest country and one of its smallest. There are approximately three million residents, and it is about the size of the state of Maryland. Moldova was once a part of the Soviet Union and gained its independence in 1992.

On my journey through the Peace Corps, I experienced many insights and life lessons. I did actually have a rooster in my bathroom for a brief period. Of course, there were many wonderful life lessons learned in other parts of my life as well, with or without the rooster.

As you journey through life, not only do you learn things, but you get great reminders from things learned in the past. Sometimes these reminders come on a timely basis, and sometimes they arrive a bit slower. These reminders certainly help because there is always so much to remember from life, isn't there?

The learnings from the past may be adapted to the changes and experiences one is going through. Part of my time in Moldova was spent with outstanding youth that I had contact with via visits to schools, attending special programs, and being involved with some unique projects.

One student who kept crossing my path both literally and figuratively was Liviu. Liviu was a high-school student who had a lot of passion for life and learning. He had many goals and was keenly interested in a variety of pursuits. He was a virtual sponge, soaking up ideas even in English, which was not his first language. His other languages were his primary language of Romanian, and Russian, which is also spoken by many Moldovans.

One cold Saturday afternoon, I crossed paths with Liviu as we were walking on the sidewalk going in different directions. It was a day of moving from one meeting to another activity for me and for him as well, as I discovered. When I first saw him going in the opposite direction, I thought perhaps I was going the wrong way or was missing some unique opportunity. However, we were both headed to different programs in opposite direction, and both were great pursuits. It was good to know there were several valuable programs and meetings that day. Sometimes things were so busy you were lucky you did not run into yourself going in more than one direction.

When you enter the Peace Corps and reach your country of service, you ring a bell to note your arrival and the start of your experience. About two years later when your time is up, you ring the same bell and are essentially ringing out and ending your time. The bell is located at the entry to the Peace Corps offices. The benefits of the memories and experience will continue through your entire life; however, you are ringing out as a changed individual. You are now packed with treasured memories; some good, some not. You realize you are filled with many lessons and life learnings from experiencing life in a different culture and being in a different world far out of your comfort zone.

The expression I came up with that worked for me to describe the daily experience was "Moldova … no day is perfect, but every day is perfectly interesting." In essence, that was very true.

Between those two bells were a lot of perfectly interesting days; a lot happened over those 27 months. Just as many things occur in one's life from birth to death, many are ordinary, and some are extraordinary.

Just like the *"dash,"* meaning that little space that represents the line between your birth year and the year you move to heaven, certainly a lot happens in that space of time. It is so much more than a placeholder or a punctuation mark. Much is experienced day-by-day all along the way.

On my ring-out day from the Peace Corps, I met Liviu at a coffee shop and soon discovered this was much more than a simple chat. As he sat down, he opened his notebook, took out his pen, and asked me for the meaning of life and life lessons all wrapped up in about 30 minutes. Liviu feverishly took notes, and I talked as fast as I could, not knowing what thoughts might spill out next.

So, if I had more time that day, I could have shared other stories and advice. In writing and publishing this book, I share stories with a lot more people than one teenaged youth. Sharing our stories is significant for all of us, whether in a verbal or written format. These stories may naturally be the passing along of moments and lessons to your friends and family. Sharing stories adds to our humanity.

While I spoke to Liviu, I encouraged goals and lifelong learning. I focused on exploring as many things as possible and not to be afraid to try something new. There is the only failure in not trying. Of course, many of the things that don't turn out well become the chief learning experience to prepare for something else down the line. Many times, we won't even realize that until years later.

Reflecting on that conversation that August afternoon in 2015, if I had more time the last day in Moldova, I could have told more stories and shared more life lessons. My life has been an interesting one, and a creative one with many unique experiences.

I served in the Peace Corps and was active in the entertainment industry in Hollywood as a playwright, theatrical reviewer, performer, writer, speaker, and more. While in Los Angeles I worked in advertising and had opportunities to work in video, print, radio, and television. Yes, that degree in Mass Media and Communications from the University of Akron eventually paid off.

I had more than 500 articles published in newspapers and magazines and co-authored a few books. I performed standup comedy at the famous Ice House in Pasadena. I was on stage with Joan Van Ark, Lee Meriwether, Lainie Kazan, and Debbie Reynolds.

After my advertising job ended, I switched gears by taking training to become a hypnotherapist. You learn many things from "unemployment," but I call that "getting your new freedom to do other things in life." Advertising can be a quick turnover industry, and I was lucky to hang in there for 16 years.

Somewhere in the middle of all this, I survived the Northridge Earthquake even though I lost my car which was flat as a waffle iron, dealt with my condo that became rubble that fateful day in January of 1994 and lost lots of stuff; for sure, everything breakable. Things can break of course, but this does not mean that one is necessarily broken. You can bounce back; what great lessons one can learn from a disaster. At the time, the earthquake seemed devastating -- and it was. In reflection, though, it was just another journey in life's marathon.

We never know where life will take us. You might one day be sharing your bathroom with a rooster. Yes, this is nothing to crow about. I do hear that roosters have a morning personality and seem to want everyone to have a morning personality as well. On the other hand, it just might not be so bad, and there is often humor in nearly every situation. Life is your personal marathon. So, let's start Section One and the first chapter with lessons learned from an actual marathon: the Los Angeles Marathon.

"A journey of a thousand miles begins with a single step." This is a famous quotation from Lao Tzu, the ancient Chinese spiritual leader. So, let's step out, shall we?

Table of Contents

Section Three:
Peace and Pieces

Section Four:
Special Pets, People, Places and Things

Section Five:
And One More Thing

Section One

Hooray for Hollywood and LA
LA Land

Chapter One

LA LA Land, Running Elvis and Dead Toenails
(That is not the name of a Rock Group)

I had a goal to complete an entire marathon, and that meant all 26.2 miles of it. I think this is a popular goal on many people's bucket lists, and yet not so easy to accomplish. You do have to get off the couch and engage in the process and stay involved. Just thinking about it won't do.

Step-by-step I completed the Los Angeles Marathon in March of 2005. Unlike marathons such as the Boston Marathon, which has certain requirements for participants, the Los Angeles Marathon takes all comers. And I do mean all comers.

When you see guys (and even gals) next to you running in Elvis Presley costumes, including blue-suede shoes, you pretty much understand that all-comers' concept. The Los Angeles Marathon is a colorful, rich cultural experience as you meander throughout numerous neighborhoods with the aromas in the air serving to identify a dominant ethnic food in an area. Entertainment and treats are plentiful along the way as you hit the pavement step-by-step in truly one of the greatest cities in the world. Thousands leave the starting gate, plugging along mile by mile; not everyone makes the finish line. There are the serious runners, those running with a goal, and there are those participating just to be in it and have a great time. When you hear Randy Newman singing, *I Love LA* at the start of the race, you are ready to love the experience of a marathon winding its way through LA-LA Land. And, you truly love LA in one of its' finest moments.

I soaked in the sun and dealt with sunburn, waved at the running Elvises, and made new friends along the way. Just as in life, your running and walking mates continually change throughout the day. I received a wrong number calling my cell phone and chatted with this woman about what I was up to in the marathon and what was going on. Somehow even though my phone rang she thought I had called her. From wrong numbers to lots of side shows it is a day of surprises, challenges, and personal growth.

I dedicated each of the 26.2 miles to someone or some specific thing, and I prayed along the way. I walked each mile and reflected as I did it. Once you get into the miles in the twenties, things get tougher. The miles seemed a little longer. Actually, they seemed a *lot* longer. It always helped to see the next mile marker in your sight, as it gave a better feel for how far you must go. Sometimes when a mile included twists and turns, you could not see the next mile until you came very close. In life, it is easier to view your own goals as mile markers that are in sight for you as an inspiration and a reality, but even when you might not be able to see the next mile marker, your spirit needs to move you on the way.

The day went along, and I got increasingly tired. When the race officials removed the traffic barriers after the faster runners concluded a segment, slower runners and walkers had to adjust. You are still going, so you need to be aware of vehicle traffic, and you may need to move up onto the sidewalk. There are then no free passes through traffic lights, so that may slow your pace. You just have to wait, like all other pedestrians. Yes, they do have pedestrians in Los Angeles. These changes provide a reminder that even when you are on course in life, things change, and you need to adjust and re-evaluate continually.

There was a younger man I partnered with for a segment of the race. He was having difficulties. He had no problem letting a woman help him out. Dropping your ego is a wise decision during a marathon. At some point, we were no longer connected; I moved forward, and he took a break. This occurrence happens in the marathon of life as people come and go, and some are just with you for a time or a specific experience and others are there for the long haul.

At some point deep in the route there was a sign that said, *"What Were You Thinking?"* and you can laugh, or you can cry, but better to grab for some deeper resolve that you were planning to finish and that is what you are going to do.

After 26 grueling miles, the final two-tenths of a mile comes into view.

Pretty soon you begin to see all the decorations at the finish line. It seems both close and far away. The final two-tenths was easy and hard. I was excited that the long journey would soon be over. As I was crossing the finish line, I phoned my mother in Ohio. Crossing the finish line, I was draped with my medal and other items and you are celebrated even though thousands crossed the finish line before you. It truly is your own race. Just as your life is your *own* race.

I met my goal of finishing while reflecting and soaking in the experience. Special thanks to the volunteers and all the people who cheer you along the way; that applies in life as well as a marathon race.

I was exhausted. It was a good exhaustion. I felt completely drained. I was happy to complete a major goal.

I was thankful I had taken the train that morning because I would never have been able to drive from downtown Los Angeles after the race. That morning when I boarded the train to come to the race, I had wondered if other marathoners would be on the train. As I got on the train, it was filled with marathon participants dressed in their marathon shirts, so it is like the event started right there, with everyone talking and sharing in the pre-race moments as the sun began to rise over Los Angeles.

As I was composing myself after the race and trying to figure out where the closest train stop would be, a woman offered me a ride. I was grateful to be driven back to the San Fernando Valley to pick up my car at the train station. On the way, we talked about the experience. My driver was planning to participate in the future and wanted to begin to setup a plan for participating in the marathon. I had not been in a special training program, and I think that was something she seemed to want if she registered. Her goal was to make it more of a journey of several months before the race and training with other people. In my case, I shared my experience that I increased my walking and visualized what it would be like to be in the marathon. I had participated in 2004, to soak up the feel and learn about the marathon while completing a half-marathon, to follow with the full race the next year, trudging the entire course. Each runner has their own goals for being in the race. Some are just in it for the fun of the start and the perks along the way until they drop out. There is nothing wrong with that.

Happy to be back at the train station after I was dropped off, I was barely able to handle the short drive home. It seemed long since I was so exhausted. It was only about a mile. The marathon was on a Sunday. I managed to have extra energy Monday and Tuesday and then was exhausted on Wednesday. You notice your dead toenails for the next several days after finishing a marathon. I was warned about this. It just seems to be part of the process. Lose a few toenails, gain grand life experience. That is a good tradeoff. It was a great journey, but I have no desire to do it again. Some things seem more special if you do them just once.

Some lessons from the marathon that also apply to the marathon of life are to dedicate yourself --and prepare for the journey. Sometimes others will be there on the way, and sometimes you are on your own. Either way, make the most of it, and ultimately it is your own journey.

Some of those along the way will be good for you and others won't. You may be good for some and not as worthy for others. That is part of the life journey. Appreciate those who help with your life journey. Celebrate your victories and the victories of others. Keep going, as there are always new miles in the voyage of life.

"The secret of getting ahead is getting started."

Mark Twain

Chapter Two

A Little Bit of Hollywood—Rolling Out the Red Carpet

I was fortunate to produce the Red Carpet Awards in Los Angeles. The event was associated with Women in Theatre, a local non-profit. I served as president of that organization. I became the creator, producer, and emcee at the Red Carpet Awards. This was an awards program to honor all the elements of the live theatrical arts. The awards included not only actors and plays, but puppetry, poetry, props, publicity – just mentioning some of the "p" words, plus anything and everything that has to do with live performance. As far as I could research, there was not an awards program like this anywhere in the country.

My vision was to bring together a theatrical community in Los Angeles, which is probably the most diverse and productive city in the world. LA does not have the Broadway blockbusters but has many big productions. However, the landscape of Los Angeles is decorated with many small theatres that devote themselves to everything from opera, children's works, play readings, comedy, interpretations and more. It is spiced by the extensive range of culture in the community, plus people's passion for the unusual.

It was especially lovely to honor organizations or individuals who helped those with disabilities, or the underrepresented and those who strived to do new things. Back behind the scenes is where the real work gets done, not just on the stage. There are so many who handle such a wide variety of details. I appreciated learning more about these crafts, which can be very creative and require a lot of talent, as well as dedication.

One year, we honored Jim Maurer, who played a baby grand piano voluntarily in the lobby at St. Joseph's Hospital in Burbank to help inspire and entertain patients and hospital visitors. Singer Melissa Manchester was his award presenter. A lovely backstory is that Melissa and her mother Ruth would take a break and go to the piano recitals when Melissa's mother was a patient at the hospital. Lo and behold, Florence LaRue of *Fifth Dimension* fame was also a presenter that same year and had also enjoyed Jim's talents on the piano when she visited patients in the hospital. She mentioned this as she presented awards to other individuals. I got to know Florence when we both served on a theatrical judging panel; that's when I asked her to be a presenter. It was so inspiring to note these connections. It shows how much art reaches people and its impact -- even in a hospital setting.

In year two, actress Joan Van Ark was our official celebrity from the Honorary Board of Women in Theatre, which included numerous well-known individuals. Joan became sort of a godmother for the awards by coming back to be a presenter, and she submitted nominations as well.

Joan had a great deal of diplomacy and was a caring and cooperative spirit. She shared stories about her Hollywood experience when I talked to her. While she was working on *Knots Landing*, Joan started her day with Debbie Reynold's brother, William Reynolds, who did her hair and makeup. How one starts the day can affect motivation. Sure, to some it may seem to be a thrill to be on a national television show. But the early calls and long hours and issues to deal with can also take a toll on anyone.

William not only did her hair and makeup but got Joan motivated for the day ahead. It would be nice if we all had someone like that, wouldn't it? If you don't have someone regularly, you will have to do it for yourself, but it is nice to have a motivator or an inspirator, and there are many resources for that, if not an actual person.

Years later, we honored Debbie Reynolds with a Red Carpet Award, and Joan graciously returned to pay tribute to Debbie by being her award presenter. I was selected as well with an award, and it was nice to share the moment with Debbie Reynolds and other awardees.

One year, Michael Learned, who played the mother on *The Waltons,* attended the event. *The Waltons was* a delightful and inspiring story of a family set in the early 20th century that was a popular television show in the 1970s. She was very warm, charming, and complimentary in our brief conversation. She went out of her way to talk to me. We can readily engage and connect with people and at least on occasion, go out of our way to do so and share a compliment or a good thought.

Picking up the phone one day I heard, ...*Please hold for... Lainie Kazan*. I think I must have always imagined getting a call from a celebrity preceded by those words -- Please hold for....

I did get calls from celebrities, but generally, they had called me on their own without a lead-in from a member of their staff. Upon receiving the call from Lainie's staff member, I quickly accepted and had a lovely chat. Lainie was to be an upcoming recipient at the Red Carpet Awards.

It is always nice when you are producing something of this nature to be able to do exceptional things for someone. My brother Dennis was a fan of Lainie back in his teen days. He had even gone to see her perform when he was in high school. I offered

Dennis a slot on the entertainment program. He was a solid and inspiring singer who had done solo shows, been virtually the only "white boy" in a gospel choir and had even sung a little backup for songstress and composer Melissa Manchester. He was thrilled to perform and did a fabulous job. Lainie Kazan enjoyed hearing his story of seeing her on stage, and that added to the moment.

It is funny how life comes full circle in many ways -- even more so if you pay attention. I encourage you to seek the occasional daring goal, find ways to honor others and do something special. Occasionally, call yourself and say...Please hold for...you! Who better to take a call from? Make sure you share something magnificent.

"The greater danger for most of us lies not in setting our aim too high and falling short, but in setting our aim too low, and achieving our mark."

Michelangelo

Chapter Three

The LA Scene -- What's on Stage and on the Radio?

Once in a college writing class in Ohio, we had a guest speaker who was an entertainment reviewer. I thought *I would like to do something like that one day.* Many years later, one of my friends in Los Angeles contacted me to let me know that a local newspaper, *The Tolucan Times*, needed theatrical reviewers; she encouraged me to contact the paper. I was interested but thought I had enough things on my plate. She then called me a second time at work and prompted me once again. Thinking about that day in my college class and not knowing when the opportunity might ever present itself again, I contacted *The Tolucan Times* and went in to chat with them. It turns out you can always add just a little more to your plate, so I did.

I soon received my first assignment, which led to a few hundred other articles and deadlines for more than 13 years. This was freelance with the emphasis on the free if you get my drift, but it opened several rich possibilities and great opportunities in the wonderful world of theatre. I met a lot of creative and dedicated people. There were even those who requested that I be their reviewer and I had some fans who mentioned they liked my columns. It was nice to hear that when someone said that to me as then, I knew people enjoyed the theater columns.

There were a few times I did not want to go to a show, but of course, needed to go anyway. It could have been the weather, or I just did not feel well or something else. It was on those occasions that often I was especially won over. So, the performers had not only won over a reluctant member of the audience but also gained a big fan.

One of these occasions was *Opera Works*. It was a warm Sunday afternoon, and I think I may have wanted to enjoy the weather rather than being stuck in a theatre with "stuffy" opera performers. However, I was in for a big surprise. *Opera Works* delivered a menu of opera on many levels, and it was anything but stuffy. It was comedic, creative. and a breath of fresh air. The performers did a lot of shticks while maintaining their operatic bearings, which is hard to do. One skit was about a performer subbing on a roadshow for a performance. The individual may have the music down cold and can do it to perfection, however blocking is always a bit different, depending on the venue and other factors. The performance of this concept was brilliant and led to many laughs. The performers did their opera magic while bumping into each other and missing prop calls and more. It was delightful and put my day-at-the-beach thoughts into cold storage.

Another memory is of a performance staged Elvis style. Just imagine *Hound Dog* mixing with Puccini, and you note the contrast and possibilities for great humor. The energy, the timing, and the talent needed for all these performances was incredible. *Opera Works* has been very successful for decades in greater Los Angeles and beyond. *Opera Works* was an honoree for the Red Carpet Awards and well deserved, I might add.

It was a dark and stormy November night. I was feeling dark and stormy as well. I had not asked anyone as my guest to attend a festival of barbershop quartets with me. I was not excited about listening to barbershop quartet performances for two hours, and it was the only chance to go, as it was a one-night show.

I think after two groups performed, I was clearly won over by the creativity of each performance and its specific style. A few years later, one group, *The Valleyaires* -- now known as *Valley Harmony Chorus* -- was honored at the Red Carpet Awards for their longevity, charitable work, and dedication to the craft of barbershop-style singing.

As a theatrical reviewer, I met a lot of people who added immensely to my social life and life experience as well

One night I attended a play and just could not get into it. The story was being told backward, and that was annoying me. After about 20 minutes, I converted from being bothered to starting to recognize brilliance. I began to appreciate the writing and how it was being portrayed. After about 40 minutes I thought that this play could be nominated for an Ovation and in fact, it was. The Ovations are LA's version of Broadway's Tony's, on a smaller scale.

The play *Hello* was written and directed by Stefan Marks; he and Beth Patrik starred in it. Yes, in fact, it did garner several well-deserved awards at the Ovations. One note: sometimes you must give some things and certain people a little more time to see the brilliance come out.

Lesson learned: there are diamonds in the rough that don't exactly pop out like diamonds at first glance, but you need to hang in to uncover the jewel. That applies to people, as well. You have probably experienced people you were not that impressed with on first meeting but then discovered some excellent qualities and talents.

There was a production that I attended called *Burn*. *Burn* is a one-woman play, a searing journey to personal freedom and transcendence; the coming-of-age of a little girl locked in a desperate struggle with her mother for sanity and love in a post-WWII German Displaced Person's Camps. I came to know Ingez Rameau, the performer/writer of this commanding play, and even sent her an email suggesting that this show was strong enough to be done off Broadway. And, in fact with my encouragement and I am sure the backing of many others, she did take the show to New York.

Speaking of Broadway and off Broadway, I had a distinctive opportunity to interview director Charles Rome Smith in one of the back offices of Theatre West in Hollywood.

Theatre West is a classy theatre with a variety of programs and has been in existence for several decades. I made several friendships at Theatre West. Barbara Mallory and Lloyd Schwartz produce plays as part of Storybook Theatre at Theatre West. Lloyd wrote and produced *The Brady Bunch*. His father, Sherwood Schwartz, created the show. Storybook Theatre won a Red Carpet Award for its dedication to young children's stories. Dina Morrone, my favorite Canadian, even though I have never heard her say "*eh*" is a producer/actress/writer who has served on the board at Theatre West and staged several productions there. Plus, Dina was a tremendous help for the Red Carpet Awards. If you don't have a favorite Canadian, you should get one. Canadians just seem to be really nice. Garry Kluger is a member and prolific playwright there as well. He also received a Red Carpet Award and offered graphic assistance for many years for the event. Theatre West is a great place with wonderful and talented people.

My normal pattern as a reviewer was to see a play or a performance and write a review of about 250 words. Interviewing Charles Rome Smith as part of the publicity for an upcoming show at Theatre West was a nice bonus and a change of pace as I was conversing with someone and not just reviewing a play. This time was a pleasant opportunity to have a conversation with someone and get into a long chat about experiences in show business, including Broadway and off Broadway.

I still had just the usual 250 words. But we sort of whiled away the time at Theatre West talking for hours. The focus of my article was to be on an upcoming play Mr. Smith was directing. Beyond that, it turned out to be just one of those nice conversations that reflected many special moments of life and the arts on a Saturday afternoon.

For me, it was a few great hours of wonderful conversation and connection conducted in the back room of a legendary local mid-size theatre while almost feeling the spirit from the nearby Hollywood Bowl and the theatrical scene in Hollywood. I left our talk feeling very satisfied and happy. Reflecting on my desire to be an entertainment writer back in my college days, I felt pleased that I had a chance to do this type of writing, paid or not. I was getting my rewards in other ways.

I was excited to write about a variety of people in a multitude of roles. Sometimes there is too much concentration on the acting. I always remember a great line: "The scenery was terrific, however, sadly the actors got in front of it." It takes a village of talent to do lots of things in life, including a theatrical production.

Ahh ... radio. I had majored in mass media and communications while in college, which was a perfect major for me. I had an opportunity to start my short radio show at American Radio Network in Hollywood -- and produced it as well. That just sort of means you pay for it. But it sounds nice, doesn't it? You may get sponsors to pay the cost of production if you can.

Each 15-minute show featured a couple of commercials and a few songs. I was partial to Motown, the Beatles, and standards from Perry Como and Frank Sinatra, but the music was quite varied. Each show also included a life lesson. You are probably getting a few of these by reading this book, so don't feel bad if you missed the broadcast. The topics could be related to health, education, goals, making the most of your life, and more. At that time, I had completed training in hypnotherapy and did a short segment about the use of hypnosis to improve one's life which usually was a theme of that show's special topic.

It was great to be on the radio and have the creative flair for doing my own thing while manning the audio board broadcasting. I received several compliments about my voice and writing abilities. However, I did not receive much hypnosis business from the radio show. I merely chalked it to the fact that I did something I enjoyed, and this further connected me to the media. I was fortunate as a senior in high school to be one of the high school beat reporters on a local radio station, talking about teen activities and events. It was a lovely opportunity for me as a teenager. I never thought that later in life I would have my radio show, broadcasting from Los Angeles. It was fun while it lasted.

I stretched myself by doing something new and improved my voice for my hypnosis clients while being on the radio. I had a chance to be creative, improved timing, flow and much more. There are always opportunities for growth in everything you do.

Take advantage of opportunities and try something new. Find ways to express yourself and enjoy all the moments of life.

"To become truly great, one has to stand with people, not above them."

Charles de Montesquieu

Chapter Four

A Whole Lot of Shaking

The 1994 Northridge earthquake occurred on January 17, at 4:30:55 a.m. PST and had its epicenter in Reseda, a neighborhood in the north-central region of the San Fernando Valley in Los Angeles. It had a duration of approximately 20 seconds (it seemed longer), had a magnitude of 6.7 and produced ground acceleration that was the highest ever instrumentally recorded in an urban area in North America. The death toll was 57, and about 8,700 were injured. Also, property damage was estimated to be between $13 and $50 billion, making it one of the costliest natural disasters in U.S. history.

January 19, 1994 is a day I will never forget. My condo in Reseda was just a short distance from the epicenter, and my complex was along the Los Angeles River, so the ground was softer than other places. There were plans for bike trails and more along the river that would make the community even more engaging and active. After the earthquake, these plans were scrapped, just to get the neighborhood back to a workable level. All these years later, this development has never happened.

I had been through many earthquakes in Los Angeles, as they are frequent. But there was never anything like this one. The quake put out a noise that sounded like a train crashing. The shake was so dynamic that I thought it might be the end of the world. I discovered several of my neighbors had the same thought.

A woman's loud, chilling scream pierced the early-morning hours. I was sure someone had been killed. No one in my complex died, nor did I hear about any serious injuries. Chatting with other neighbors later, we never found out the who and why of the scream. It was likely just from utter fear. However, that moment was scary and overpowering in a way I had never experienced before.

When the quake hit, I was thrown about a foot-and-a-half into the air from my sleeping position. Shortly after the initial quake and numerous follow-up aftershocks, I looked out the window and saw that it was pitch black. Not a light in sight anywhere, as all power had gone out. No working traffic lights, or street lights; everything was just dark. It was a darkness I had never experienced before in an urban area. You could not see anything.

The damage to our building could not be determined before daylight; we were a couple of hours away from the dawn. From the start, it is likely that part of the complex fell on my small car parked underneath and it was flattened to be just inches in height. Large and smaller tremors continued, and when the light came, it was easy to see the damage to the building. The tremors were persistent as the morning went on. I looked at the rear of the building continually collapsing, and it was almost as if this were a movie. I was in disbelief. How could this be happening?

It was surreal to look out and see your building falling. It is as if you are caught in a dream. Your hard-fought aspiration to buy a condo was collapsing; this was your home, and the buildings were the homes of others, as well. I was trying to tell myself that things were not so bad but felt alone and unsure. About 11 a.m. the fireman came to say I had five minutes to leave.

What to say? What to do? No car. No phone availability. What do you take?

A bit earlier when the inevitable seemed to be happening, I contacted my brother, Dennis. Phone service would be available for a few minutes on landlines and then would stop. I was able to connect with my brother Dennis who lived in the East San Fernando Valley, and I lived in the West San Fernando Valley, about 10 miles apart. Dennis was reluctant to come to pick me up, and I don't blame him, but he did anyway.

I took some things to a nearby storage facility. Because their computer was down, they did not want to rent me a unit. The family at the storage facility lived in an apartment in the storage complex and since they were so isolated did not have a feel for the extreme damage in the area. Some places really looked like a war zone.

I explained that in a few hours their facility was likely to be filled up, as people would begin to take things from their homes and need to find storage. I was just the first of many, and they needed to expect an influx of business over the next few hours. I asked them to do the rental the old-fashioned way, without computers. They rented me a unit, and we worked out details later. And yes, by 3 p.m. all their storage units were filled.

Later I found out that one of the men who worked at the facility had a heart attack. Heart attacks are not unusual in these types of circumstances. The facility had a stressful situation that did not just end that day but continued for several weeks.

Staying in North Hollywood at my brother's apartment, I was notified that my employer, Precision Dynamics Corporation, had the foresight to seek some hotel rooms to help people out. I did receive one of these hotel rooms for a few days. That helped me to think, relax, and sort things out. Save for a few travelers who unfortunately did not have the best timing in booking January in Los Angeles for a vacation; the hotel was filled with relocated earthquake victims.

People were completing insurance forms, lamenting the loss of family heirlooms and keepsake items with significant memories from deceased relatives that were now smashed to pieces.

My refrigerator was jostled around and developed a chirp like a bird. When I had relocated, I joked about it for a while when people came over and heard the chirp. I then mentioned my "bird." One day when the chirping stopped after I had purchased a new refrigerator, someone asked me what happened to my bird. I said I did not have a bird I had a chirping refrigerator. Oh, the lengths you'll go to have a pet.

The Northridge Earthquake was the best of times and was the worst of times. It brought out good things in people. They helped. They encouraged. They served meals and pitched tents for people.

It also brought out the worst in people. Some tried to get funds to which they were not entitled. Some stole things. Some people took advantage of the situation and people who were stuck in tough circumstances.

When a city the size of Los Angeles is struggling from a natural disaster, this can influence the whole country and the world; California has one of the top economies in the world. Work went on to get things moving and repaired. Some things happened quickly. Other efforts took a long time or were never fixed.

I had paid an extra premium for earthquake insurance. This is complicated to explain; especially with several condo buildings sharing certain things as well as being separate entities. However, insurance payments did help me with some incidentals and moving expenses; however, I soon would be paying a mortgage plus rent for an apartment, which was a huge challenge. Investment in some earthquake coverage was money well spent even though the actual building and that loss could not be covered. However, my small earthquake coverage was like winning a very tiny battle in a gigantic war.

One day a few years before the earthquake, I was watching television and people were evacuating their homes due to some disaster. I don't remember if it was flood, fire, or hurricane; however, I remember thinking to myself what a terrible position to be in. What a way to make the national news -- and then one day I was one of those on the national news. I was not interviewed, but some people said they saw me on a broadcast covering earthquake damage. We were right at the epicenter and photos of my condo also made national publications. My condo was the "cover girl" for the *Los Angeles Daily News* magazine. Just when you think you can get away from it, you make the front page. People moved out, and yet there were a few hangers-on who probably did not have anywhere to go or the resources to handle that. It is not easy and takes lots of effort.

My condo had been switching from a co-op to a condo for some time. This was an expensive legal process, yet I assumed this eventually would work in my favor. However, because of the earthquake, it did not.

The condo transition had recently taken place, and then I was able to refinance from a very high-interest rate to a lower rate, thus lowering my housing expenses, which were a huge part of my income. The property would have bumped up in price in a year or two, as well. I had paid considerably to get the new loan, and it was only refinanced for a few months. So, bottom line, I had put out a lot for little return and was never going to realize the advantage of lower payments and a boost in the market.

What I owned was a pile of rubble, and I had a mortgage payment and now had to pay rent on top of that. How crazy is that? How could I go on with that sort of burden?

I learned a lot from experiencing a big disaster. The Lord giveth and the Lord taketh. The "giveth" part always seems much better.

To help out, I visited one of the tent camps where people were staying. I was grateful and glad that I went. I was in a bad situation. However, these people had it much tougher. There was little privacy. Dealing with small children and babies who do not understand what is going on is a challenge. There is confusion about what will happen next. Not only did some people lose their homes, but on top of that lost their jobs. Many decisions had to be made soon and more in the future.

In America, many live in standards the rest of the world only dreams about. We tend to expect more and may complain about the smallest thing. There are millions throughout the world where food and water are not easily attainable.

While staying at the hotel, I overheard a phone conversation where a woman was complaining about losing some of her favorite beauty products -- and her spa was closed because of damage. This was in sharp contrast to many other issues of real survival.

There were many perspectives from the earthquake. Some people were merely inconvenienced. Some were not hampered at all. Some had the ultimate loss of life. And others lost their favorite cream rinse.

The Lord giveth and the Lord taketh. About three years after the earthquake I bought another condo in Toluca Lake. Toluca Lake was one of my favorite areas of Los Angeles. Yes, there was a lake, but I never saw it. My condo in Toluca Lake did appreciate over time, thus taking away some of the stings of my earlier traumatic loss.

There were people who lost not only their homes but apparently may have lost their job in the earthquake as well. I remember listening to broadcasts wondering if my employer's complex had been damaged. I found out soon that things were okay there although some reorganizing was going on. There have been people in Southern California who got hit with catastrophes of more than their share — fire, flood, mudslide, earthquake and who knows what else. I heard of someone who experienced three such disasters in a few years. It makes you wonder.

Surviving and thriving from a disaster may take a while, but with a little good fortune, it can be done. You come out a stronger person. You also learn the Richter Scale is not the one you have in the bathroom. Each little number adjustment marks a huge difference.

Faced with a major or minor disaster, be aware and get a true perspective. Be thankful for what you do have and be prepared to switch gears. Stay in community and vow to bounce back, even if it takes a while. You can always use your personal Richter Scale in life. When it goes up a little, it means a lot.

"No matter how bad things are, you've got to go on living, even if it kills you."

Sholen Aleichem

Chapter Five

Still Shaking

There are often many issues that crop up in the aftermath of disasters. In the early fall of 1994, I became quite ill. I had never been this sick before. There was a sort of virus that many people who were earthquake victims seemed to pick up at about the same time. It may have been stress, breathing in the toxic air from smoke and asbestos from falling buildings and other factors. I was having troubling breathing, was constantly wheezing, would cough so much I was throwing up and many other symptoms, some of which I have now forgotten. I stayed in bed. I missed more than a week of work. It was difficult even to get up and prepare something to eat. A year later I was still experiencing some of these same things, such as coughing so hard I was throwing up.

Many people have medical and health issues after undergoing major tragedies and upheavals. Just about the time, all these things had started to fade; I was driving by a medical clinic for women in Burbank. As I drove by I experienced a strange sensation in my left breast. It was like the heat was generating. This served as a wakeup call and as a reminder that I should get an exam.

Soon after I scheduled an appointment, after the doctor had my X-rays, he called me into his office to show me there was a large tumor as big as a tennis ball in my left breast. It would need to be removed by surgery and done in the hospital. As I understand, some women can have lumpectomies of smaller tumors within a doctor's office. However, this was not the case in my situation.

I scheduled surgery at St. Joseph's Hospital in Burbank because I considered it to be a great hospital. Prior to my surgery, a short, older nun entered my room. With 12 years of Catholic education, I quickly sized up that she was not carrying a ruler, and all was safe. She was sweet, and we said some prayers.

Soon I received some papers to review and noted a word I was not expecting. MASTECTOMY! No one ever used that term with me, and nervously I asked to see the nurse. She soon came to explain. As I understood, because of the large size of the tumor it was classified as a mastectomy and not a lumpectomy. However, I was reassured the tumor would be removed, and nothing else was going to be cut off. However, this procedure was considered to be a mastectomy -- a word that could be misinterpreted.

As I awoke in the recovery room, I was attached to several machines, but the other patients seemed to be lying quietly in a bed without all this paraphernalia. I was informed that I had to stay awhile as I had stopped breathing during surgery and they had to bring me back. I think this is not so unusual, but not a regular procedure. They needed to monitor my vital signs, so I had to stay longer than expected. After having the sounds go off when I wasn't breathing enough, I got it worked out and did the required time without having any more warnings sounding. I kept the nurses on their toes until I was able to assure the alarm was not going to go off anymore. During the surgery, I felt I had that moment of going down the tunnel that many people experience as a near-death moment and then sort of was sucked back in. It was all very vague. It just had seemed weird to me as far as I remembered. It was somewhat inexplicable, and we will leave it at that.

My mother had come from Ohio a day before I was in the hospital. I asked the staff not to say anything about this extra incident to my mother, and soon after some struggles with doing the required breathing I was breathing okay, and I was released.

I was startled that my body was a little different than expected and it would take more than a year for everything to straighten out. Even simple things, like opening a car door, were tricky and it took me some time to adjust. The good news was that the tumor was not cancerous. I have a long scar that I must explain at medical appointments. So that is not so bad at all.

My mother stayed with me for a few days. Initially, I felt she did not need to come from Ohio, and it might be difficult for her. However, the next morning after the surgery I had great difficulty getting out of bed and was so glad she was there to help me.

Going through disasters or tragic incidents brings out the awareness of the need for empathy and understanding. Many times, we oversimplify incidents or undervalue their impact especially if they have no direct influence on us. We are familiar with the Golden Rule "To treat others the way you would like to be treated." A stronger approach would be the Platinum Rule which is "To treat people the way they wish to be treated." Yes, sometimes that is difficult to do, but it is beneficial to figure out as you need to go deeper to understand people.

After nearly three years post-earthquake, I was out of the woods on the health issues and had purchased a new condo, gotten a raise, and a promotion. Life moves on.

"Keep your face to the sunshine, and you can never see the shadows."

Helen Keller

Chapter Six

Sleep with Me and Wake Up Your Life — The Power of Hypnosis

I had always been interested in the mind and how people think. I noted adjustments that we all can make to provide clearer thinking and increased insight. From the time I was a small child the process of hypnosis fascinated me. It could add clarity, provide change, give focus, and serve as a beneficial form of relaxation.

Sometimes the Vegas-style hypnotic shows where people pretend to lay eggs as chickens, do wacky things, and act in a highly humorous manner have served to define hypnosis. However, those are conducted for entertainment purposes in highly suggestive situations; sometimes, alcohol helps.

Hypnosis and hypnotherapy can make for lasting change and move lives into remarkable and improved situations.

After getting my new freedom to pursue other things in life (losing my job), I enrolled at the Hypnosis Motivation Institute in Tarzana, California. I began to study hypnosis in a year-long diploma program. During the internship phase, I was required to log numerous client hours to fulfill the graduation requirements.

Studies completed; I began my hypnotherapy practice after graduation. Getting clients was a challenge, but the help I provided people was highly rewarding. There were many surprises in working with clients. They often presented specific issues to work on and yet received what I would call a "by-product" that helped with other matters in life as well.

Some of the Best Stories

I worked with a client who had performed on stage for years. However, after a long career, she had developed stage fright and was reluctant and uncomfortable to go onstage. We worked on the issue in office sessions, and as a bonus, I went to one of her performances and did a brief hypnotic session for her in the ladies' restroom just prior to the start of her performance.

It all worked very well. She had renewed confidence, which showed in her singing and instrument playing. She had fun. The audience had fun and was entertained.

It worked even in some different and unexpected ways as well. I ran into her at a neighborhood event just two months after our final session. She had met and married a man she liked who was a good fit for her. I should mention she was in her sixties and not a rebellious twenty-something. She was also more confident and readier for life's next step. The hypnosis had provided these extra benefits to her.

Another mature woman was seeking something in her life that yet had not become apparent. She had written a laundry list of issues to work on. Some were related in many ways, and others were more distinct.

In one powerful imagery session, I was surprised by the results. *M*, as we will call her, had received a strong vision and had a desire to paint artistically. She had never noted this passion before the session. Surprisingly, that very day she enrolled in an art class and began painting. She painted and painted some more, virtually non-stop for three weeks and then her art went on display in a gallery for a showing. . Now, those are some tangible, life-changing results. She was very grateful and had a much more defined meaning to her purpose in life. Growing up in a large family in Europe that encouraged the pursuits of boys and ignored the wishes of girls, she had moved into her truer self as a middle-aged adult.

M was very grateful and had a much more defined meaning to her purpose in life and looked at life on a larger scale than ever before. The hypnotic process had led her to a new way of life on a journey to success.

Another client, *S*, was seeking something but was not quite sure what that was. In her second session, a surprising result appeared. She decided she wanted to share her life story. Her family had a history of mental illness issues that influenced all the family members. Her 60th birthday was just a little over a year away. She decided to tell her story in a play that she would write and perform. Taking this on was quite a goal from someone who had never done anything like that before.

She quickly got some acting training, direction, and writing coaching. She stayed dedicated to her mission and concentrated on her goal, much to her credit.

The result? A year later I was sitting in a theatre in greater Los Angeles watching her deliver a thought-provoking show. What is remarkable in all of her efforts is not only had she received the vision of this program in the hypnotic session, she also gained the motivation to follow-up with an action plan to get the right resources, appropriate people, tools, and a venue to make this dream a reality.

It is often difficult to know the impact that can be extended to others inspired by the story and the journey. We never fully know what may transpire in their lives and their relationship with others by discovering a story and hopefully acting on it. Every match, when lit, starts with a small fire that can ignite something else and produce tremendous energy.

Another example: Our mind's viewpoint can influence our perception of pain. I worked with many clients who were able to eliminate and/or reduce physical pain by going through the hypnotherapy process. One client who worked a night shift sent me an email after she had completed her midnight shift, expressing that she was able to go for a long walk for the first time in ages. Her knee had been giving her constant pain, and now the knee was more fluid. The pain was reduced, and she took a long walk during her lunch break in the middle of the night. She had not been able to do that for quite some time. This was a great success for her that led to other things, including weight loss, increased exercise, and satisfaction.

I worked with a teenager who had the opportunity to play varsity baseball for his school, moving up from the junior varsity. However, he was struggling at bat and in the field. After the session, he told his mother he felt it was a waste of time. However, the very next day he had the game of his life. He completed some spectacular defensive plays in the field and was hitting the ball well at the plate. He was won over with the hypnotic process and came back for other sessions to work on other issues. For him, hypnosis had been a grand slam.

It was a privilege to help people increase the quality of their lives via the hypnotic process. It was inspiring to witness transitions both large and small that allowed clients to be healthier, wealthier, and wiser. I would say every client gains in some way even if it is just to become more relaxed and open to new thoughts and possibilities. Hypnosis can be an intensely spiritual experience. Most of us go to a dentist twice a year to care for our teeth. I think seeing a hypnotherapist or similar professional a couple of times a year is a great idea to gain a life purpose, overcome issues and gain clarity in addition to working on specific challenges at other times.

Sleep with me and wake up your life was a phrase I used as a tagline. It is fun, of course, and a nice play on words. However, the hypnotic process often referred to as *sleep* can change lives positively in so many ways. I encourage you to question and explore your thinking, find ways to make the most of your life and help others to maximize their existence as well.

"No day is perfect. Every day is perfectly interesting."

Trish Ostroski

Chapter Seven

Reflections on 9/11

I am working on this book, and it is September 11, 2018, as I write this. I think this marks an appropriate ending for this section regarding Los Angeles and Hollywood. I am reminded of another great story. Let's go back to 2001.

In August 2001, I attended a breakfast for San Fernando Valley Leadership at the Beverly Garland Hotel in North Hollywood. I was privileged to have been a participant in this organization's signature program. There are many of these leadership programs that follow a similar plan with collective experiences held in numerous cities throughout the country. Actress Beverly Garland, well known for her appearances on the television show *My Three Sons* and many others, had also been a participant in the program and the organization's events were frequently held at her hotel.

Coming into the event I saw Marianne Haver Hill, who was the CEO of MEND (Meet Each Need with Dignity), an outstanding service oriented non-profit in Los Angeles and sat with her. I soon discovered that sitting right next to me was Bryce Zabel, newly elected Chairman/CEO of the Academy of Television Arts and Sciences. He was the speaker for this breakfast.

Bryce and I had an in-depth, though brief, conversation on leadership until it was time for him to speak. One of my specific questions was regarding being placed in uncharted territories and responding with grace and true leadership at the moment. I doubt that he even remembers this. However, the memory stays with me because of the events that would soon transpire on September 11 and the repercussions that would follow.

The September 11, 2001 attacks (also referred to as 9/11) were a series of four coordinated terrorist attacks by the Islamic terrorist group Al-Qaeda on the United States on the morning of Tuesday, September 11, 2001.

The Emmy Awards, traditionally held in September, were fast approaching on the Sept. 16. Discussions ensued about postponement and whether to even have the event at all. No Emmy Award presentation had ever been canceled. This, of course, had an impact on CBS, the Academy, the venue, the people and numerous other factors. The reality during those turbulent days was trying to define what was "appropriate" and what "tone" the event should take in an entertainment landscape as well as the country reeling from the impact of the attacks.

The awards were rescheduled to October and then again moved to November 4. It ended up being broadcast opposite the World Series as the New York Yankees dueled with the Arizona Diamondbacks. The dress code moved from formal to business. The two months change in the time allowed the show to inject some humor in the situation. Ellen DeGeneres balanced the inclusion of humor while maintaining a respectful tone. In the interim between the attack and the airing of the show, Bryce Zabel demonstrated excellent and crafted leadership to do the right thing when no one knew what the right thing was.

The night of the show, Phil Driscoll's trumpet solo of "God Bless America" opened the show and, later, Barbara Streisand's "You'll Never Walk Alone" ended it, thus creating a start and finish in a proper perspective for the night.

Host Ellen DeGeneres struck a perfect tone with timing that was spot on. Addressing thoughts regarding the terrorists who had attacked the USA just two months earlier, she said: "They can't take away our creativity, our striving for excellence, our joy," she said. "Only network executives can do that."

Customarily, the Chairman/CEO of the Academy of Television Arts and Sciences has a brief spot on the television airing of the Emmys, and it is usually not a highlight moment. But Bryce's presentation the night of the show was memorable and impressive. Additionally, it had me thinking about our conversation of just a few months before. Who knew that after that August breakfast there would be such dramatic changes to consider? He was ushered into his office as no one ever has been before. Here is a quotation from his speech on the night of the awards.

"Terrorism doesn't stop with shattered glass and shattered lives. It aims to crush the spirit of the survivors. To have given up (on the Emmys) would have been more than a postponement or a cancellation, it would have been a defeat. That's because for fifty-two years previously — through war and peace, through assassinations and civil unrest — the Emmys have been awarded on television. Like baseball and Broadway, we are an American tradition. Especially in such challenging times, these cultural touchstones become important. Many millions of viewers from more than 90 different nations are watching tonight. They see us exercising our freedom to assemble, and proclaiming that fundamental ideal that inspires all artists, freedom of expression."

As I was watching, I thought of our conversation at the August breakfast and how especially the thoughts we exchanged were strongly prophetic. I doubt that Mr. Zabel would even remember talking to me. However, I remember that moment.

There are two lessons here. The first is to get out in your community and take advantage of talking to people. Yes, it can be challenging to put yourself out there, but there are many rewards to reap.

Secondly, we must strive to do the right thing in leadership, and we may not know for sure what that is. We have observed many scandals and cover-ups, and these exist because people are afraid to act or feel they don't know what to do. To do nothing is the biggest wrong. Once you take a step, other steps begin to reveal themselves. The people who may criticize you are doing nothing, and since you have put yourself in the moment, as Bryce did, you know more of the overall situation.

"All that we are is the result of what we have thought; it is founded on our thoughts and made up of our thoughts. If a man speaks or acts with an evil thought, suffering follows him as the wheel follows the hoof of the beast that draws the wagon.... If a man speaks or acts with a good thought, happiness follows him like a shadow that never leaves him."

Gautama Buddha

LA-LA Land

I was thankful for all the experiences I had in Los Angeles. The opportunity for creativity and the ability to meet people who want to accomplish many things is probably unparalleled in any other city in the world.

My life path wrapped around there and was enhanced by many experiences there and other places as well. In Section Two we explore Life Paths including goals, learning, and the meaning of life.

Section Two

Life Paths

Chapter Eight

The Right Time to Lose Your Job or How to Go on a New Life Path

Shortly after I made my final payment on my earthquake loan, which took several years, I was laid off from my job. I had a co-worker who was continually fearing her job loss. Currently, with mergers and acquisitions, it pretty much seems to happen to most people at some point in their life. A merger, a move, a new product comes, another product goes away, sales are up, sales are down. These events all influence the economic cycle. Sometime, take a look at companies that years ago were on the Fortune 500. Few of these remain intact today. Circumstances change, and the business world adjusts its course.

My co-worker thought they would never let *me* go. I knew this not to be realistic. Besides I worked in advertising. It is not unusual for people who work in that field to be forced to change jobs because of advertising agencies switches, new products in and old products out. It happens.

I had told her there is not a good time for this to happen. However, it would be nice if all the cherries lined up for a job loss or what could be called *How to Go on a New Life Path.*

It would be nice if you put the maximum amount in your 401k for the year. In my case, that had just happened the previous payday. It would be nice to have the max amount of vacation. That day I had also achieved the max in vacation days, and the account freezes till you take a day off. However, I would soon have many vacations days. Third cherry to line up was to reach a certain amount in my 401k. That had just happened on that day as well. Three cherries all lined up. It was time to go on to other pursuits. I think God was moving me along.

It also was nice that this was just before Thanksgiving and I could have some more leisure time over the holidays. Since there was not a real rush to get back from Ohio to Los Angeles at Christmas time, I took the train for the return trip home. This was something I had always wanted to do. From coast to coast the train just moved along. I watched the passing scenery and was lost in my thoughts as the train chugged along from the heart of the Midwest across miles and miles to Los Angeles.

Here are some good things I discovered about my transition. You have a lot more freedom in what funds you place your retirement money once you are no longer with a company. Most companies select a certain number of accounts for 401Ks. However, after several months I kept my retirement account with Vanguard but began to explore other funds in their portfolio. At that time, one worked out very well for me. Of course, there is no certainty of that. But you are given more freedom to handle your own money, and that was a plus.

In this transition, you can explore new things and ideas. It is important to note that not everything will be a bullseye. But the exploration can add significantly to your personal growth and possibly even your professional one.

Take time to look at your life from various angles: not just professional, but also personal, spiritual, health wise, and more. Perhaps whatever you did previously became a prominent part of your identity, and you may need a new way to define yourself. Remember, work is what we do; it is not who we are. We are all many things beyond our job title. Seek a few things that will fit in with your current flexible schedule.

Go to the gym. Join Toastmasters International, a speaking and leadership organization. Read some helpful books. Catch up with friends and family you may not have seen in a long time. Read a new magazine and a different newspaper.

Are you in a rut? Challenge yourself to pursue a new adventure. Perhaps zip-lining. Only the first step is scary; the rest is terrifying — just kidding! Take on a new sport, try yoga, or reconnect to an activity you have not done in a while. Deep inside, you may always have wanted to reinvent yourself. Now you have the chance. You have received an official invitation. It might help you to visualize this invitation with your name on it. You can fill in the inside of this invitation in your imagination

Change your language regarding your former employee right away. It was us, and now it is them. Perhaps it is time for that cross-country train ride. Volunteer at your child's school. Learn something new on the computer. This stuff is always changing, or something new crops up and it is wise to stay current with terminology.

Go on a spiritual retreat. Build a ritual of prayer/meditation into your daily routine. Avoid gossip and concentrate on constructive things. What is something you may have wanted to do in the past? Perhaps the time may be right or soon will be. When I was walking out the door from my former employer, the Peace Corps flashback appeared in my mind. What might you still have a fire for even from your childhood or youth?

Change something about yourself physically. This could be new hair color or style, new color or item in your wardrobe, a different style of shoe or find a favorite thing that you used to wear that will give you comfort.

Redesign or decorate one of your rooms Even a paint job with a new color can add some zest and a new perspective. Take walks and notice little things that you never see while driving. Drive a different way down a new street or walk or ride your bike on these streets as well. Plus, on foot or a bike, you may discover some new paths on which to venture.

In Peter Pan, the advice to get to Never Never Land was to "think lovely thoughts." So, take that advice. Get hypnotized to reveal something within you. Act like a teenager for one night with some of your friends from your teens. (Be sure to get your parents' permission.)

Have a long giggle session. Roll all over the floor laughing. Watch Lucy and Ethel wrapping the candy on the candy factory assembly line. Cut things you can from your budget and your life; you will discover there is a lot you can cut. Think of it as adding, by subtracting. Take on living a bit more simply to add some extra grace to your life. Get a coach. Select a good one. Take a good hard look at your bucket list.

You can best manage transition periods by simplifying, opening yourself to new possibilities, and re-evaluating while rejoicing. Begin to create and be sure to laugh a lot.

"Beware of missing chances; otherwise it may be altogether too late some day."

Franz Liszt

Chapter Nine

Finding the Meaning of Life

I began graduate studies at Gonzaga University, a Jesuit school in Spokane, Washington. This would be primarily an online degree in Organizational Leadership. I had a longtime goal to get a master's degree, and the actual subject matter was not as important. I felt this degree path was a good one, since I always admired the Jesuits as educators, even though I had never been taught by a Jesuit or ever attended a Jesuit school. Plus, it was online, yet had an in-person campus component. In addition, there was a chance for some international study. I took advantage of this by taking a class in Italy one summer; my mother accompanied me on this journey.

My mother attended many of the classes with me and went on tours with the group. We went to Florence, Rome, Pisa, and Sienna and had a great time exploring, learning, and of course eating pasta.

I had hoped for my mother to see the Pope. He usually came out on a balcony at noon on Sundays. However, the Pope was out of the country while we were there. My mom did get a chance to attend Mass at St. Peter's Basilica and we sat directly beneath the dome and watched the College of Cardinals enter.

It was a high note for me to have my mother at St. Peter's Basilica in Rome and looking up to the dome at that moment. It was something indescribably special. In her eighties at the time, my mother was a real trouper in taking in the whole trip. A fun memory is that while we were under the dome of St. Peter's I was feeling a spiritual high to be there with my mother as the College of Cardinals marched in with their bright red robes. My mother nudged me and explained that they did not do this cardinal march at her home parish in Akron, Ohio; her comment brought the moment into a new reality.

The Gonzaga program was a good mix of social justice, ethics, and philosophy and had a touch of the arts incorporated into the curriculum spiced with a healthy dose of self-reflection. That is something the Jesuits seem to do best.

I had a few friends ask me what I was going to do with this degree. Well, one thing I was going to do was to discover the meaning of life. I felt that I needed to get to the core of what life was all about. It had probably been staring at me for many years and yet I could not come up with a way to describe it to people like Liviu or anyone who might ask or who I felt my benefit from having a deeper understanding of the meaning of life.

Drum roll … What is the meaning of Life????

The meaning of life is … another drum roll just for effect … TO CREATE!

How had I not ever come to that definition years before? It answered the question and was so simple yet so true. God certainly paved the way right from the start with those Six Days of Creation (with no coffee breaks and no union rep), followed by the day off to rest. God created everything and set the example for us. So simple a definition and yet I had never stated it in this manner until I was in the Gonzaga program.

Creativity had always been important to me, and many people considered me to be highly creative. What can one do by being smart, resourceful, overcoming mistakes to make something grand and new are all great skills? I am surprised I never came up with this definition of the meaning of life before my grad-school experience with Gonzaga. But there is a right time for everything in life, and I guess that was my right time.

I found TO CREATE to be the best answer for the meaning of life. So much must be created, from human life to nature, to artistic endeavors, peace, friendship, humor, fun, and relationships. Just think about anything. It must be created. Good will, trust, responsiveness, plans, hopes, dreams, good thoughts, bigger thoughts, taking in the whole of things. Yes, everything needs to be created.

Look around the world. Roads, schools, traffic lights, parks, ideas, college majors, gardens, computer programs, non-profits, awards, scholarships, directions, beauty products, clothes, laundry hampers, cleaning products. Someone had to create it. Our very existence and our ability to get to a higher existence depends on our ability to create, as well as everyone else's ability to create.

Writing this part of the book at this moment, I am creating something that never existed before. I am participating in a Tom Bird Write Your Book in a Weekend Workshop. I am plugging away for more than eight hours a day and step-by-step pouring my book out along with about 100 others who are attending the class in person or taking it online.

Think about that virtual concept for a moment. It is certainly on the newer end. For centuries, we have gone to school in person and taken classes with the instructor in the room with us. Think just a moment that someone had to come up with this idea to even start education in the first place. It is of more recent vintage to take classes online, sometimes live and more often at your convenience. You can tune in across the time zones, to attend via your computer, laptop or phone for a class going on somewhere else in the world. Imagine the creation that is coming out of this class. Creation not only for the author or speaker, but for others as well.

This book is a creation for others who may read it as well. Readers may engage in it, think about it, be reminded of something, be entertained, perhaps read something that will be life-changing, or start a new idea or a new movement.

The mind is never in the same place as it was the day before or even an hour before. This is creation. TO CREATE is a continuum.

For example, think about the birth of a baby. What a creation that is. Life comes together in a matter of moments yet gets scripted over a lifetime. The people they encounter, the work they do, how they serve the world, what they contribute, just being there, the effects on the economy and more. We all have meaning for other people, and we need to do a stronger job of protecting that and recognizing that.

In our world of tweeting instant comments of no real communication value, dishing others to make ourselves seem more important, living in our silo, we need to be reminded to get in touch with our creation that builds for others.

I admit I think that somehow, I was going to get something extremely profound such as a prolific paragraph written by a great philosopher for what the meaning of life is. Instead, my answer was two words and eight letters. TO CREATE summed up the meaning of life so succinctly and yet it is so true and encompasses so much.

Do you have a response to the meaning of life? If not use mine and see how it works for you. Is your response easy to say, workable, encompassing and true? If not, use mine and see how it works for you. Is your response ground into your soul and your being? If not, use mine and see how it works for you.

Explore the meaning of life, and be sure to create and come up with your meaning of life. After all, you only get one life. This is not a dress rehearsal.

"One does not need to travel the world, read every book, or ponder every thought to discover the meaning of life. All one needs to do is to create."

Trish Ostroski

Chapter Ten

Goals and Learning
The Non-Hitchhikers Guide to the Galaxy of Learning

I remember as a small child a few of my siblings, and I were walking to Catholic Mass. We never hitchhiked but were often given rides by people going in the same direction.

One day a family of a dad, mom, and two children offered us a ride as they were going to church as well. After we got in the car, the dad was discussing that once an individual had received their First Communion and Confirmation, he did not see the need for further religious instruction. These are both important spiritual milestones.

As a child, I was somewhat shocked that he felt this way. I thought there would always be more to learn about many things in life, especially spiritual issues. There would always be things to be reminded of and held in a deeper perspective as I got older.

That is the day I decided to be a lifelong learner. This gentleman gave us a ride; however, I took his limited perspective to be the impetus to be sure to always take the ride of my life as far as learning new things. Sometimes you get good advice from people, and sometimes you get bad advice, and you need to analyze this as a child even if you are getting information from an adult.

I find this learning to be especially true in the spiritual arena. One can always get a deeper understanding, and we continually are in different perspectives due to age, circumstances, and life experiences. From that point for me, at around ten years old, I was on a journey to be a lifelong learner and always pursuing something new. If someday down the line I offered a ride to some children, I wanted to have something better to tell them.

While in the Peace Corps, I studied Romanian and while not being particularly skilled at it, the study did open my perspective. I continued to rise in levels of understanding in the language even though I was hardly an expert. Primarily, my jobs were with English-speaking organizations and youth who wanted to improve their English. Consequently, I did not practice and use Romanian as much as some others in different language circumstances. So, you do have to be sure to practice and use your skills when you get the chance to help yourself improve.

Currently, I am taking violin lessons with an international organization called New Horizons. It is designed to help build musical skills for adults. Many are refreshing themselves with instruments they have previously played while others are playing an instrument for the first time and learning basic music theory. I am in the latter category. This pursuit is good for your brain and provides a different group of people for friendship, as classes are conducted in a group.

Participating in this program has led me to notice the string section of orchestras and little details of their performances. Each instrument is its own little world, and yet all of them put together make for a wonderful blending. Each adds to the whole. I sometimes enjoy practicing, and sometimes I would rather be doing something else. I can see the joy and appreciate the understanding that music adds to one's life. Take a moment and just imagine what life would be like without music and or sound. It would be drab and barren without life's soundtrack. What do you think?

Life offers so many opportunities, and we are fortunate to be around in a time when you can get details and facts with a few clicks. Pretty amazing. Approach life with a sense of wonder and you will be a walking inspiration to yourself and others.

Abraham Maslow, the psychologist who created Maslow's hierarchy of needs, did not list "inspiration" on his scale for life's basics and beyond. But the need to be entertained and inspired is within all of us. Just think when you read a brilliant quote, hear an inspiring sermon, enjoy a meaningful story, and have other experiences that inspire you what a change that makes in you mentally and physically. What a feeling!

Going to varied seminars and training opportunities is a great way to put yourself in a special uplifting program at least once a year. You will be around highly motivated people, learn new things, gain additional perspectives, and make some new friends. We all can get stuck in doing the same things over and over. A fresh training can fine-tune your life. We tune-up our cars, get checked by our doctors, but often don't give that same attention to our mental processes and our inner mind.

Remember Peter Pan and his "lovely thoughts?" What exactly is a lovely thought? We each may define it differently. We need to go to new places in our minds and hearts and help people experience a superb life journey. Keep that up, and that should create an abundance of lovely thoughts.

God intended great things for us in His creation. A word of advice — what you promise to yourself can come back to you when you least expect it. So, make some good promises to yourself that not only will enhance your life but the lives of others as well. After all, there is always something new, and learning is helpful for your brain. You never know where the learning journey might take you, and you will be inspiring yourself daily.

"The great aim of education is not knowledge but action."

~ Herbert Spencer

Chapter Eleven

Don't Rain on My Parade When You Don't Even Have a Baton

Sometimes as parents, guides, bosses, and friends, we may need to guide someone to a higher lesson. However, don't be a limiter.

I recently heard about one adult advising another not to send their child to a private school because of the financial considerations. Note: there are always ways to make things work. Many people move themselves to new levels when they have goals such as these. Say to yourself that other people do it and why not me? Why indeed? You can ask for a raise, but you will need to deserve it. You can seek new ways to enhance your position with your present employer, look to a new field, get a side hustle, or more. It takes some work and planning, but this also puts you in the mode of possibility. Then other options begin to come forth because of your new viewpoint.

For every naysayer, there is a *yaysayer* in the same situation getting it done. I once analyzed my position at my place of employment, reviewed comparable salaries, and presented that information. I got a considerable raise and moved into the bonus program. When I was ready to submit my amount for my salary, I added an extra thousand dollars, believing I would be negotiated down that exact amount. That is what happened, and I ended up getting my intended amount that I thought was fair. In hindsight, I should have acted sooner in getting more compensation.

When I was a freshman in high school, I traveled to the other side of town to attend school. My bus route took me through the downtown area. One day Ann Landers, the advice columnist, was making an appearance at a downtown department store. I brought up the possibility of seeing the famous columnist to a friend. I let my friend talk me out of it. A lesson learned. I had blown a chance to see a legendary advice columnist and the opportunity never presented itself again.

When there was a rock-and-roll star making an appearance at that same store after school, I was there right in front. I have no memory of what I did when I went home from school the day Ann Landers was in town. Had I attended her event, I would at least have a memory of seeing her and perhaps learning something from what she said.

I grew up in Akron, Ohio and we had chances to see celebrities that one might not expect from a mid-sized city in the Midwest. Each year numerous celebrities visited, such as Dinah Shore, Pat Boone, and the Cartwright Brothers, who rode in from the Ponderosa, the ranch from *Bonanza* a hit television show. They all came to town for the All-American Soap Box Derby. It was such a slice of Americana but had an international flair, as racers from all over the world arrived in Akron to drive their handmade cars down the hill at Derby Downs. I attended the parade that welcomed the celebrities to Akron many times. Special thanks to my mother who first told me about it. I took advantage of these special moments. Missing Ann Landers was a lesson for me.

So, be sure to have a spirit of adventure and take advantage of opportunities as they present themselves. Do something special regularly.

Explore something you have never done, something you have not done in a while or something off the beaten path. There is not a lot of traffic on those unbeaten paths. Keep your inner weather forecaster in focus and only use rain when it is needed.

"Do unto others as they would like to have you do to them."

The Platinum Rule

Chapter Twelve

Jump Right In—The Ice is Not Cold

It is often a great idea to project yourself as actually doing something or being something. Better yet tell people that you are doing a certain thing on a specific date; that ties you into action to make that happen.

I was taking a class in stand-up comedy to perform at the legendary Ice House in Pasadena. I had long wanted to give this unique challenge a try. As you approach the Ice House, you see the names of a wide range of performers who did gigs there. Jerry Seinfeld, Robin Williams, and Ellen DeGeneres are just a few of the names displayed. The Ice House transitioned from a folk-music club in the 1960s to a comedy club established in the late '70s.

As I was walking up to the Ice House on the evening I was performing, when the celebrity names came in to view, I thought that those individuals have performed at this popular comedy destination and now it was my chance.

While taking the class, I was projecting myself to be on stage on a specific night in December. So that alone encouraged me. I kept telling everyone the date of my performance; a few dozen friends came to laugh and cheer me on as well as to enjoy the other performers. I delivered many laughs with a cooperative audience and got a lot of kudos. It took a little courage, and it was so much fun.

One of my co-workers, Susan Farrell, even took on the role of my "manager." She volunteered to sell tickets to co-workers. That was a task I dreaded and was so happy that she took the initiative to do that. She was in sales, after all, so she was practicing her craft. She sold a lot of tickets, and I got other people to come as well.

You have 15 minutes to perform. I kept some notes on a stool on the stage in case my memory faded, and it did. When you go on stage, you are somewhat blinded by the bright lights that focus on you, and I had never actually had a chance for a real dress rehearsal. Things went well, though. There were unexpected laughs, and some expected laughs did not materialize. I threw out some candy at one point, and it ended up hitting someone. They did not sue me, however.

I froze a little bit when it was time to leave the stage, as the lights were a bit bright for me to see the steps. But they were there. I got a big round of applause at the Ice House. And the next day when I came into work, I walked in to the sound of applause.

This was a challenge I pursued, and I did perform some standup when occasions popped up for me. I got some free sodas for pay, and that is hard to budget to pay the bills, but completing this goal was a great feeling of accomplishment and joy.

Jump in and enjoy the moment. Feel appreciative of others who have gone before you. Laughter is great medicine.

"Youth is happy because it has the capacity to see beauty. Anyone who keeps the ability to see beauty never grows old."

Franz Kafka

Chapter Thirteen

Goals --- How Do You Get There if You Don't Know Where You Are Going?

First, make sure you verbalize and write down your goals. But it is not just enough to write goals. You need to have steps and a plan to make them happen.

Sometimes the goal angel surprises you, in that some opportunities just pop up at the right time and find their way to you. I did have a goal to write a play. I then discovered a chance to submit it for a women's play festival. The script just came pouring out of me. This was for a short play -- which helped me timewise, but still, I did get it done

In fact, at one arts festival where one of my plays was staged, they brought all the writers on stage for a panel discussion. One by one they asked us how long we had worked on our piece. I felt a little sad because the writers were saying like two years, seven years, etc. When it was my turn I asked not to be hated, then told them that the deadline for submission was August 15. I sat down and wrote the play on August 14 and then edited and submitted it the next day.

I did have the idea and theme in my mind for a while. When I sat down to write everything was flowing, and the dialog seemed realistic. I had the play within me. I just needed to get it on paper. We all have things within us. We just need to work out how to get it out. Some of the plays were published online before the event. It was nice to discover I had some fans who had read my play before the event; some sought me out to ask me questions. It was a great experience to go to the festival and share with other artists and fans for varied media.

The play was a short one, and that helped me complete it in a day. So that certainly helped. However, you can break things down and get part of a goal completed, especially if you have goals in your thoughts. So, write your goals down, stay active, and look for possibilities.

"Everything in moderation, including moderation"

Oscar Wilde

Life Paths

We meander our ways through life taking this road and that one to meet our goals and gain new life experiences Some special pieces of my life path involved being in the Peace Corps. The next section includes stories and lessons from that journey.

Section Three

Peace and Pieces

Chapter Fourteen

Childhood Dreams

I had become interested in the Peace Corps as a teenager saying, "Someday I am going to do that." People often think of Peace Corps volunteers as being young college graduates. However, there is no age limit and Peace Corps service has been popular with the baby boomer generation, of which I am a proud card-carrying member.

After a job loss that I preferred to call a new opportunity to go on and do other things, the Peace Corps came back on my radar. I began to study the organization and find out as much as possible about it. I waited until what I felt was the best time for me to apply -- even though there is never actually a "best time."

On June 2, 2012, I was walking home from the gym and felt the time was right to pursue the Peace Corps. I was at the now-or-never point. Upon my return home I popped on my computer and noted the Peace Corps website said they would be shutting down applications in 16 days for technical updates to their system. *Probably a marketing ploy, I thought*. However, I began my Peace Corps application, which included multiple parts and several sections.

On the deadline day, I was completing my last section of the application with the television on in the background and the Los Angeles Lakers hard at work on another victory. And on June 2,

2013, one year to the day I was walking home from the gym, I was in Philadelphia for stateside orientation with 50 other Peace Corps trainees bound for Eastern Europe and the country of Moldova. With the hope of *Drum bun,* meaning *"safe travels"* in Romanian, and with tons of luggage in tow and some people wearing multiple layers of clothes as a strategy to bring more stuff, we were off on a great adventure.

Entering the Peace Corp is quite a process. Several parts of the application included references, essays, goals, personal insights, and more. There were health and legal clearances, plus an in-person interview.

A few weeks after my interview, I received a letter that assigned me to Europe, and the community and organizational development program, with a spring departure. These were all things I wanted. Of course, this was not always guaranteed. In most cases, the cherries do not necessarily align so easily. Many people go to different geographic locations, are given a different sector to work in from their preference or expectation and may receive an entirely different reporting time than initially provided them.

Most Peace Corps volunteers go to Africa, and only a small percentage serve in Europe. Europe was my personal choice, though I said I would be willing to go anywhere. I had only voiced my preference in my mind. But, sometimes that is a good thing, so the universe knows what you are thinking.

During the process of going in, being in, and coming back from the Peace Corps, I heard from many people who also had considered joining the Peace Corps. They were impressed that I went in, stayed for my entire tour of 27 months and overall had a great experience.

Life is not easy in the Peace Corps, and there are many challenges including cultural, physical, mental and spiritual. It helps to stay on course and keep engaged. When something did not work out, I switched gears and went on to something else. My little motto was "Moldova—no day is perfect, but every day is perfectly interesting." Come to think of it, that probably applies to other things in life too. The ugly stuff fades in memory, and the good things grow larger over time.

My first Christmas in Moldova I was injured in a trolley accident a few days before the holiday. I had to stay in a Peace Corps medical facility for about a week. It is a bay of beds in the upstairs of the Peace Corps building, and when the doctor is in, she might check on you. On Christmas, everyone had the day off except for one security guard, and I was alone in the facility. I made sure my room was warm, and that was probably the highlight of my day: no presents, special treats, and no one to talk to. I spent the day reading whatever inspirational material I could find in the Peace Corps library. No trip to join other volunteers, as I had originally planned. Days like this can be tough, but they pass.

Entering the Peace Corps was challenging. Returning to America was much more challenging. This is hard to explain, and many people have been surprised that I made that statement. In being away for more than two years, you have adjusted to a different lifestyle; a varied culture, and I was rarely in a car, which is something most Americans are in every day.

Moldovans were much quieter, more mannerly and very respectful as a whole when compared to Americans. I was shocked to note the behavior in America. It took me a while to get used to the different styles of handwriting, street signs, procedures, and much more. There were references I did not understand. In some cases, these were something that was new or became more popular or prominent while I was overseas such as a product, phrase, expression, television show or another reference. A lot can change in two years.

Plus, I had the challenge of going to Ohio after my Peace Corps service. Though I grew up in Ohio and visited many times while I lived in Los Angeles, there were many new things I did not know about the area. People referenced things as if I should have known them such as stores, streets, and other places.

I had a fall on my return trip which led to a very severe wrist injury. Also, I missed a plane due to a crazy can driver, got lost with another cab driver who turned what should have been a 15 minute trip in to one that was 90 minutes and along with many challenges on that trip back, I returned ill and injured. Broken luggage, visa issue, being held at customs, well a disaster for every day. So, taking on all this new stuff was a bit shocking. Entering a mega supermarket was a shock to the system. For example, I had a choice of a couple of kinds of cereal in Moldova, and in the states, the supermarket probably has a couple of hundred, especially if you consider all the little variables even in the same brand and products. Many volunteers note the contrasts on their return to the states. The Peace Corps does provide some training, however, so this wouldn't be too shocking.

On another note, in a way, I think I was preparing to serve overseas since childhood. When I was in the fifth grade, I attended a Catholic school. In geography class, there was a sort of cartoon in the textbook. It depicted a child from the Soviet Union at the blackboard in a school classroom. On the board the teacher had written in large letters — THERE IS NO GOD! The child was crying deeply, with tears streaming down his face. That drawing stayed in my memory throughout my life. In that childhood moment, I wondered what life was like for young children in the Soviet Union. Little did I know that one day I would be a resident in an area that was once part of the Soviet Union.

It is interesting to note that when Moldova became an independent country -- though with the shadow of the Soviet

Union still on it -- the language changed overnight. One day it was Russian, and the next day it was Romanian. When children arrived for school, all the materials were posted in Romanian. The city of Chisinau came to the forefront as the main city and capital in this "new" country -- which was really thousands of years old.

After a training period of about two months that included language, culture, and technical programs, the Peace Corps volunteers receive a site assignment that would be their home and duty station for two years. There is a special tradition associated with this in Moldova. A map of the country is displayed in chalk in a parking lot. Cities and locations are noted, and there are marks for places where volunteers will be going. Per the announced plan, no one was going to be assigned to the capital city of Chisinau.

I was hoping to get an assignment close to the city, as I felt I would do better there rather than being assigned to a faraway small village. I was assigned to Durlesti, a suburb of Chisinau, and I would be the first Peace Corps volunteer ever to serve there. How nice that I had again gotten what I wanted and would be the first Peace Corps volunteer ever to serve in that city after 20 years of the Peace Corps being in Moldova. It was a pioneering opportunity.

I was assigned to a new NGO (Non-Government Organization) that had an emphasis on providing English at earlier ages for children and also to work on art and cultural programs for all. My Moldovan partner, Marina Ambrosi, had been an English major in college and worked as a translator and teacher. We clicked right away, and I essentially became part of her family, which included seven-year-old Cornelia and a year later newborn Demi, plus Marina's husband, Alex.

There is no such thing as only doing one thing in the Peace Corps and I was also involved with Durlesti's cultural center, another agency for children with disabilities, area schools, and many youth programs.

After swearing in, I arrived in early August in Durlesti, Moldova, and we went to work on planning a program for the Day of International Peace celebrated on September 21 each year. This is a United Nations holiday and continues to grow in interest throughout the world. Each year has a theme. We had a successful day with the children taking the lead with dancing, music, poetry, and song.

For the following year, we set about on a mission to become an International City of Peace. The International Cities of Peace in Dayton, Ohio is an organization that strives to encourage cities to make goals to become an International City of Peace by completing various objectives. While we were pursuing this project, I discovered that if we completed our mission, we would be not only the first city in Moldova to obtain this designation but the first city in the former Soviet Union to accomplish this. We would also be among the first 100 cities in the world to declare itself a City of Peace. A peace pole carved with the word "Peace" in many languages was the center of a peace park right in the heart of Durlesti. A Peace Corps grant helped to make this possible, and the city came up with donations and service hours as well to make this happen.

Helping make the dream of being an International City of Peace come to life was very satisfying to my little fifth-grade self who saw that hurtful cartoon many years before in the geography book. Life had truly come full circle for me on that one. I hope the peace pole stood for something and gave Durlesti a distinctive identity, which was sorely needed for the community.

If anyone is still drawing art for social studies books, I hope they reflect a more hopeful outcome.

On your journey, be sure to build a vision, provide hope, stay in touch with your inner child, and create excitement and meaning, as you bring people together.

"The initial step to creating a bright future is able to envision it. You must see it. Our vision is what we become in life. Vision allows us to transform dreams to reality via our actions."

Trish Ostroski

Chapter Fifteen

Blinded by the Light

As I was making my way through the entry process to the Peace Corps, I came to the last step: obtaining an actual country assignment. Because I had a timeline and needed to make plans for my condo, car, and so many other things in Los Angeles, I called the Peace Corps and asked my status. I was told my file was on the assignment desk, but they had not looked at it yet, and it would probably be about three weeks until the staff reviewed it.

Putting that aside for the moment I considered myself to be a couple of weeks away from hearing from the Peace Corps. I was a hypnotherapist in Los Angeles, having entered that field after a successful career in advertising. In LA, there seemed to be a lot of people pursuing this inspiring vocation by training in the hypnotic process.

The following Saturday, after calling the Peace Corps regarding my assignment, I had a first-time hypnotherapy client for a 1 p.m. appointment. Appointments for first-time clients generally take an hour and a half. There is a discussion of the presenting issue. The client and therapist get to know each other, and of course, there is the usual paperwork.

All of this is followed by a relaxing session in a reclining chair; the lights are brought down low, and the client leans back and gets comfortable in the chair. With eyes closed, the client readies herself to move into the hypnotic state.

I was up close to my client at first, delivering my verbal script to her, and then after several minutes moved back to my desk. There was a little rectangular mirror on the wall in the office about a foot long. The office I used was in a suite of offices that all the offices look the same with a desk, chairs, reclining chair and a little mirror on the wall. Suddenly from that small mirror, streaming lights began to shoot out and were swirling all around. It was a mixture of shooting stars and lightning and was simply astonishing. This show swirled around me, and I did not know what to think. I continued to deliver messages to my client while taking in this powerful light show in a state of disbelief.

After about a minute the light show swirled back into the mirror and then swirled out to the wall next to the mirror and gradually dissolved. Yes, I was sure this was some sort of spiritual message. However, I must admit I looked at the mirror just to be sure someone had not installed some sort of special-effects device in the office, but I knew that was highly doubtful. However, I needed to stay grounded and continued to deliver an effective script to my client to help with her issues even among this impressive light show that was swirling around me.

On the drive home from the hypnotherapy offices, I could think of little else than the bright light. Upon returning to my Toluca Lake condo, I went to my computer, and I noticed an email from the Peace Corps. Feeling a little nervous, I checked a couple of other emails and then said a prayer and opened the email from the Peace Corps. It was my invitation to serve in Moldova. Thinking back to the light, I noted that the email came in at 2:04 pm and that is exactly when the light show sparked forth. Since it was a Saturday and would have been after 5:00 p.m. in Washington, where the Peace Corps headquarters are located, the email was unexpected on that day and time. One simple email, but one that marks a dramatic life change. I had only heard about Moldova for the first time a few months prior in a presentation by a returned Peace Corps volunteer. I was surprised that it was the only European country I had never heard of and yet now would be a major part of my life story.

I felt that the light show was a message from God, and this was truly my mission to go into the Peace Corps and to this former Soviet Union country. This was a journey that had started that day in my teens when I said one day, "I wanted to go into the Peace Corps and serve." Moldova, here I come.

There were still a few hurdles to get over including double checking some medical issues and getting final approval on that. Those were worked out, however not without considerable effort. However, I began donating items, gifting things, selling a few things, and slimming my life down.

On occasion in life, you just might get a wonderful spiritual moment — enjoy it and don't try to over analyze it. Be ready to be surprised.

"When you arise in the morning, think of what a precious privilege it is to be alive – to breathe, to think, to enjoy, to love."

Marcus Aurelius

Chapter Sixteen

Downsizing -- To Throw Away or Not?
That is the Question

It is interesting that we all seem to have a lot of things we seldom use and accumulate many things. They just seem to pile up. We don't use a lot of this stuff; we would likely be better off with fewer things -- stuff that we used more -- and give more to others who might need it or simply enjoy it.

I had accumulated several awards which included plaques, trophies, statues, and some awards that resembled the Oscar, and just got rid of these things. Noting this task on Facebook, some people mentioned why I did not store these things or give them to someone to put in their home. To begin with, you are just burdening someone else and/or paying a lot of money for storage. Storage is best used short-term for transitions when you are painting or repairing your house, or other similar situations. Otherwise, you are paying extra money to store things you paid for and don't have room for. There are exceptions, but if you are hoarding or have too many things, it is wise to look at your lifestyle regarding how you handle these types of situations.

I sold my 2007 Toyota Corolla, finalizing that about three hours before I had to be at the Los Angeles Airport for my flight back to Ohio, where I would visit for a few days before going overseas. Then for more than four years, I did not have a car, relying on public transportation and keeping things simple. This included my time in the Peace Corps and a return to Ohio afterward to assist in the care of my mother until she had gracefully moved to heaven.

So that you know, Peace Corps volunteers do not have cars and are not permitted to drive. The goal is to live like the people you are serving. This includes using public transportation and living simply. As far as "going to the bathroom" it might mean using a hole if that is the only facility available. You are to engage in the culture and the everyday life of your country of service. As Americans, we are spoiled with all that we have and all that we expect. If one truly embraces the opportunities within the culture and the people, you have taken a deeper step into your soul. It is not about stuff. It is about people. It is not about bling. It is about service. It is not about your comforts. It is about comforting the world.

Concerning going to the bathroom and all the rituals surrounding that: There are many untold stories of unusual places and circumstances to take care of business that would include both number one and number two and in some circumstances number three. Those instances are classified. As I understand it, most Peace Corps volunteers after their return jot these down and place the stories of these incidents in an envelope. The envelope may be opened 50 years after their death and only if someone needs to know. Oh, the stories. Oh, the experiences. Oh, the laughter and the tears.

Volunteers are encouraged to be involved with their site city rather than continually seeking to get together with fellow Americans in their off times. Those outings are important too, and sometimes a relief, but it is essential to be an integral part of your new community, and that increases your cultural inclusion as well as the chance for the residents of another country to get to know you.

Each volunteer, even in the same country, can have a vastly different experience in living arrangements, assignments, people, transportation, and plumbing or the lack thereof. I lucked out in plumbing as I did have a modern house in which to live. However, it was not high in water pressure, and we had a lot of electrical outages. I learned from my first host family during my training period that you don't put the toilet tissue in the toilet. I was yelled at for doing so. Who knew? You learned to do things quickly as you just might be without power or water and be in a half-finished situation.

The Moldovans make such good use of materials and tools and are resourceful with gardens and animals, even if they did not live on a property that would be considered a farm. Agriculture, including the making of wine, was a main part of the economy. For a second-world country, it had solid internet access, so you could even use your computer while going to a more primitive style of bathroom. See, there is a silver lining to everything and why not, as you have learned to always have something at the ready for toilet paper. Volunteers were always well supplied with tissues in their pockets or learned to regret the lack of that. Toilet paper or tissue was never taken for granted. Having these paper goods handy is a habit that might take you a few weeks to remove yourself from after you return to the states. However, my mother always encouraged my ten siblings and myself to be sure to keep a tissue handy at all times.

We often hear of First World and Third World. I think many people do not understand what the Second World is. The First World now usually refers to Western, industrialized states, while the Second World consists of the communist and former communist states. The Third World still encompasses "everybody else," mostly in Africa, Asia, and the Middle East, and tends to be a catchall term for "developing nations." Moldova was in the Second World category, as a former communist state.

Be mindful of being resourceful, live simply, downsize when needed. Be sure to keep some tissues. You will always need them.

"Simplicity is the ultimate sophistication."

Leonardo da Vinci

Chapter Seventeen

Serendipity — How I Met My English Tutor

Peace Corps volunteers are required to continue with their language studies after the initial training period. After you are in your job, it may be easier to understand what your needs are in tackling a foreign language. Certain terms and vocabulary could be very helpful. Most of our class of volunteers concentrated on Romanian; a few learned Russian. Everyone was given some expressions and words in both languages for familiarity.

I moved to my site in early August and set a goal to have a language tutor by the end of August. I had met a young man at the post office who spoke English well. His name was Dan, and he assisted me when I determined the rules in my new post office were not the same rules as in my training city post office. We became Facebook friends

After contacting some tutors from a list and trying a few other things I thought to ask Dan about the possibility of being my tutor. He informed me he was now working in Germany, but he had a brother who might be interested. By the way, working in other countries is quite common for those living in Moldova. Many people I met had been or soon would go to other countries, separated from their families and striving to make a living to send money back home.

Just as Americans might move to Chicago or Los Angeles, Moldovans often move to other countries to work. Sadly, they often leave their children behind to be raised by relatives. It is a big issue, and the situation makes it difficult for families. A good-paying job in another country certainly helps economically. However, it leads to lengthy separations, hardships, and children being away from their parents for long periods. It was rare to note a family that did not have this issue.

Back to Dan and his brother. I did not know how to get in touch with Dan's brother. But wait. You have heard of *How I Met Your Mother*. Well, this is *How I Met My Romanian Tutor,* but you won't have to wait for several seasons to get a resolution.

I was still new to my site and the day-to-day routines that are the norm in the community. I was spending some working hours in the cultural center. This was a building that had the post office, the marriage registry, and a stage and auditorium for community programs. The toilet facilities were basically holes. Just so you note it was not modern or efficient by any means even though later in my service, a modern recording studio was built there.

I was often coming and going at the cultural center. The people were not used to me or my schedule; in fact, I did not have a regular schedule. One Friday everyone left early, but I was still working in a back office, and they probably did not realize I was there. The locks and doors can be a challenge, and you often cannot get out from the inside. When I checked the door, there was no way out for me. I called my Moldovan partner, but then my phone died. A big sin for Peace Corps volunteers – a dead phone. *Shhh...don't tell anyone.*

I began to pound on the door. The post office should still have been open. The key was in a little hole on the other side. I did not know how to even describe this in English, let alone in

Romanian. A voice answered my call and to my surprise responded in English. I said, "Oh you speak English!" The response? "No kidding." Well with a little searching my rescuer was able to find the key in the sort of crack in the wall where keys resided. *Shhh… Don't tell anyone.*

My rescuer opened the door, and there was a "Dan" look-alike with a different haircut. This was Calin, and I discovered that the brother Dan had mentioned was his twin. So not only was Calin Dan's brother but also his identical twin.

It was the end of August. I had set a goal of having a tutor by the end of Augus, and one showed up most unusually. I spent the next few hours with Calin. We visited a local artist. I went to Calin's house for dinner, and after dinner, I had my first Romanian lesson with my new tutor. When you have goals, sometimes the solution finds you.

Language studies also involve becoming aware of culture and history. Calin was full of tales about Durlesti and the surrounding community. He shared stories from Moldova's independence. For example, as a young child, he came to school the next day after independence was declared, and everything had been changed from the Russian language to Romanian. That is quite a difference for a child and of course quite a change for a new country.

One connection often leads to another. Calin was in his thirties, but he did have a brother in his teens. Duru was a bright and professional student and became a member of my Diamond Challenge Team along with one of his friends. Diamond Challenge is a competition that encourages students to write a business plan and to be able to pitch the plan and field questions. I was pleased that my students passed the written submission and moved on to the pitch phase of the competition where they would need to field questions and answer them.

Our team's project was a wedding-planning service. The students did well enough in their written presentation to have made the initial cut. They were a bit nervous in the presentation phase, and I had to encourage them, with the help of some others. Some inventive education and service ideas took the top prizes. I was pleased that our team did well enough to be in the top group that at least moved to the finals. I made a goal that next year my team would be in the top three.

That worked out, as the next year I had two remarkable boys who put together a Santa-style delivery service. They launched the business and made money. They did a dynamite presentation, including wearing Santa suits. They were up at the first rooster crow that day to practice even more. They put an impressive amount of work and dedication into this program. My goal of having the team I mentored be in the top three was met, as we placed third and the students won some cash and prizes. It was a joy to work with these boys and watch their extensive growth through their participation.

Always have goals -- and sometimes the goal finds you. Keep up your energy. You never know where connections might take you. Maintain the enthusiasm that youth have.

"Remember, no effort that we make to attain something beautiful is ever lost."

Helen Keller

Chapter Eighteen

The Color Purple

Peace Corps volunteers are encouraged to reach out to other organizations in their community. I had pretty much walked just about all the streets of Durlesti, the city in which I lived. I discovered an agency tucked away down a lane that helped disabled children. After meeting the leaders of the organization, I added this new group to my work assignments.

This agency was sort of hidden behind housing and was not easy to notice. However, their work was truly noticeable. Someone had tipped me off about this group, and I began helping them edit the English on proposals and attended special events such as parties and zoo trips with the children. For them, it is a delight to have someone from another country accompany groups. During my service, in many cases, I was the first American someone might have met. You have to take that as a personal responsibility.

Purple Day was an event in which this organization for children with disabilities was involved. The goal is to bring attention to autism worldwide. We have struggles serving people with disabilities in America. Other countries have much more of a challenge in meeting so many needs. Children with disabilities have a difficult time in any country, but even more so in second- and third-world countries. There are simply not enough resources, and many times there are well-meaning people who lack the skills, education, and experience to focus their agencies on concrete and continuing results. That is a worldwide problem as well.

On Purple Day, it was fun to meet in Chisinau at the heart of the city square. Numerous balloons were released and flew overhead. The expressions on the children's faces were precious.

I enjoyed being with the children and understanding the challenges their families, and especially the mothers, took on.

To help at the agency I wrote some reports for the United Nations. It was a good learning experience to note standards throughout the world and shared goals that link countries together. After all, this is a world we share, and something that happens to some of us truly happens to all of us.

Be sure to keep seeking and learning. Find time to celebrate and make the most of your opportunities. Gain a world perspective even from one person and even from one child.

"Wisdom is oft-times nearer when we stoop than when we soar."

William Wordsworth

Chapter Nineteen

A Loaf of Bread, A Jug of Wine, and Thou

I was very impressed with the Moldovan youth and their behavior and the respect I received when I visited schools. I was treated like royalty. I must have seen a ton of plays about chickens and other animals. The children were well- behaved and were dedicated to doing well. They get graded daily in each subject.

Because I was probably the only American living in a city of 15,000, people get to know you and notice you. They see you walking in the streets, shopping in the stores, and attending meetings. In essence, you are a celebrity. You come to discover that a lot of people know things about you and in a lot of ways you wonder just exactly how that happened.

Speaking of walking on the street, I had one lovely, memorable interaction with a teen girl. One bitter cold and icy winter day, I was walking from the transportation station carrying my very large computer. Transportation was plentiful at the main road and other places nearby, but the walks from there to where I lived was a rugged road, hilly, and goes over a river.

Walking downhill with a computer can be challenging. A girl who lives by me was also walking down the hill and offered to help. We walked arm-in-arm. One Moldovan. One American. One generation to another. A quiet walk mindful of the ice which can sometimes be a surprise. Life's slips and slides can sometimes be a surprise. This is symbolic of the Peace Corps journey as well as life's journey -- going down a rough road, sometimes having some extra weight with you, someone helps you, and you also may help them. Your time with them may be short, but it may be significant. There are bumpy roads in the Peace Corps journey and bumpy roads in life -- but you navigate, and it helps to go arm in arm. Each generation helps each other in different ways.

It is important that you engage with as many people as possible and you need to be on guard for the unexpected. I went to a high school for one event and soon found myself judging a costume contest for Halloween. I have to say the entertainment and games were impressive. The school went all out for Halloween, even though it is a holiday that is newer to them. I have to say my best and most memorable Halloween in my life was in Moldova for this unexpected Halloween party at the local school.

Speaking of holidays, one neat thing about Moldova is that it seems as if there are always two holidays for everything. Two Christmases, two New Year's and other holidays as well. There is a celebration for the holidays that might coincide with American dates, as well as Christian holidays and then also for Eastern Orthodox holy days and holidays.

Most of the country is of the Eastern Orthodox faith; however, many do not actively practice. Services generally last three hours, and you stand. There are many days of fasting and abstinence adhered to by the devout. People acknowledge religious icons even as they pass them by walking or driving by on the streets by using the sign of the cross. Entering the churches, worshippers go around and kiss and devoutly acknowledge dozens of icons.

There are several blessings for schools, classrooms, cars, and more. Icons are freely displayed in many schools. Once Moldova left the Soviet Union there was a religious fervor. There were not enough priests or ministers to accommodate this. The Eastern Orthodox church came up with a short training rather than the usual years to get enough men in the clergy ranks to serve the people. I thank my tutor Calin for telling me all about the "four-month priests."

My favorite holiday was Easter Memorial. This is held the Sunday after Easter. People come in droves to the local cemeteries for a blessing of graves. I was surprised at the number of people attending. It was beyond my expectations. While you are at the cemetery, you can see large groups of people on the route and walking up the hills.

After a long winter, this might be a time and place where you can reconnect with your neighbors you may not have seen for a while. People gather around gravesides and prepare for the priest's blessing. The deceased family members are honored and remembered. This holiday seems well placed in the calendar to follow Easter and is held usually when the weather is warming up. I was amazed by the devotion shown on this day as well as the throngs of people all over the country participating. I will always be impressed by that memory.

America does have Memorial Day, but often concentrates more on the fact that it is a three-day weekend than honoring the deceased. Of course, there are still many programs to honor fallen service members, and many people do private traditions for their family as well. These still do not have this decorum and respect that Moldovans have in their honoring of their deceased.

Large masas are common in Moldova for holidays, and special events and people get together and dine. A masa is a festive meal.

It is common to have a cold round of food followed by a hot round of special dishes. Wine is very popular in Moldova, and it is a sizable industry. There were many opportunities to try a variety of wines, and many families have their homemade stock.

In a lovely welcoming ceremony for me in my site city, children presented me with a special loaf of bread. Moldova had many wonderful traditions and rituals that were very meaningful. I was happy to be involved in these traditions and learn from history.

Be sure to honor the deceased in respectful ways to include honoring the culture. Keep traditions and start some new traditions.

"Knowledge includes the facts, information, and skills acquired through education and learning. Wisdom is the quality of having experience, as well as knowledge, and good judgment."

Trish Ostroski

Chapter Twenty

There's A Rooster in My Bathroom

Yep, this is the chapter you were waiting for. While serving in the Peace Corps in Moldova, I dealt with several bitter, cold winter days. This was a bit challenging after living in Los Angeles for many years. One winter day I heard a sound coming from the porch. It was an agonizing sound. At first, I thought maybe it was one of the dogs, as we had several. It sounded as if perhaps the animal was suffering from the cold. I went to see what was going on, but could not spot anything. On occasion, I heard the sound again. I had not ever heard a sound exactly like that.

The next day on waking up, I did not hear that same sound, but another strange one. It sounded very close, and in fact, it seemed as if might be coming from the bathroom. I got up and went to the bathroom for my usual morning ritual. Well, I had an audience. Sure, enough there was a rooster in my bathroom, sitting in a box. I was sure that was the animal generating the unusual sounds from outside, the day before.

Because I figured out that the rooster was suffering from the cold, I had empathy for it. I would want to be inside, too. Perhaps the rooster was as surprised to see me in its bathroom home as I was to see it.

If I had just arrived at my site and discovered I had a rooster in the bathroom, I would have gotten on the phone to the Peace Corps and said, "There's A Rooster in My Bathroom!" I would have been in shock and dismay. But I could see the humor and necessity in the situation.

The Peace Corps inspects living spaces for its volunteers before they move in. Though I lived in a pretty nice place, it had not been visited by my program manager in advance. She had visited another home for me and came to check the day I was moving into the place I ended up living. The community was just trying to work out something quickly for housing so that they would have a volunteer -- their very first one.

However, I could be more flexible at this point in my service and not be alarmed, while having empathy for this creature. Plus, I suspected the rooster was not long for this world. So, I decided not to complain and make its' last moments warm ones. I strived to find the humor of the situation. It made for fun Facebook posts. Besides I had no idea that I would one day use this situation for the title of this book. So that all worked out well, didn't it? I hope the rooster does not have an attorney post-mortem. Or, it is not a question of Bed, Bath and Beyond. That beyond thing has always scared me. How about you?

After about a week, I came home and saw a bunch of feathers placed together in the kitchen. The Grim Reaper had come, and the rooster I suppose would be part of a meal for my host mother, or someone else, never to crow again. I think the rooster at least left this world well-fed and warm.

There would have been a time I could have been weirded out about such an experience. Instead, it gave me some good stories.

Also, I came to get more in touch with other animals and the fact that animals in general often count on us for much of their care.

On some level, the rooster and I became kindred spirits. I think our eye color may have even been similar. Well, hey, we were roomies -- or perhaps *roosties*.

"Energy and persistence conquer all things."

Benjamin Franklin

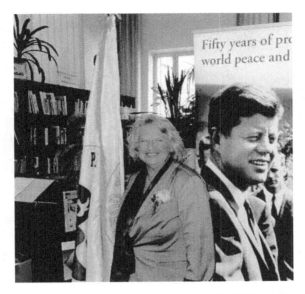

Peace Corps swearing in ceremony August 2013. This marked 20 years of the US Peace Corps relation with Moldova.

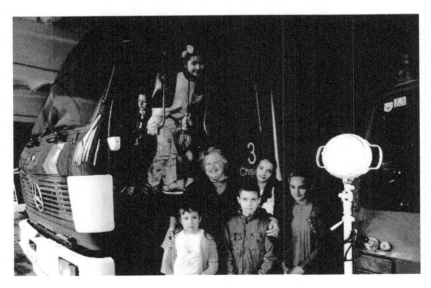

Summer camp visit to the Firehouse. Just as fun as when you were a child. The Moldovan children were always so engaged, polite and respectful.

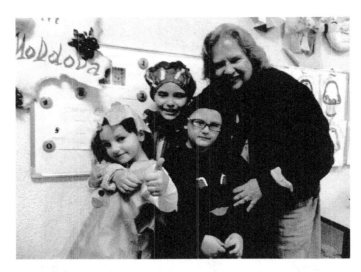

There were many festivals in Moldova. This was an autumn festival in October 2013.

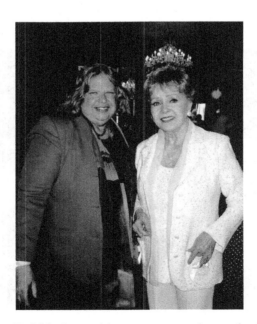

The legendary Debbie Reynolds was an awardee at the 2011 Women in Theatre Red Carpet Awards in Los Angeles, and I was humbled to be honored as well.

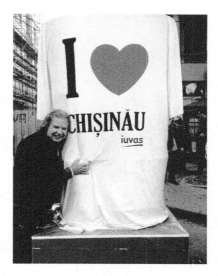

In downtown Chisinau, Moldova the capitol city for a special event. There were many adventures during my Peace Corps service in Eastern European.

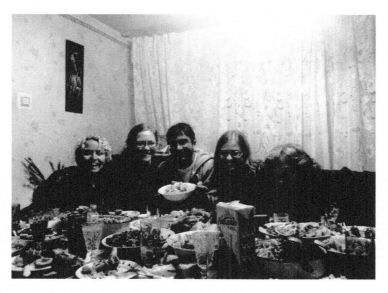

The most fun Thanksgiving ever in 2014. Peace Corps volunteers and another American share the day at a Moldovan house. So many laughs and so much fun.

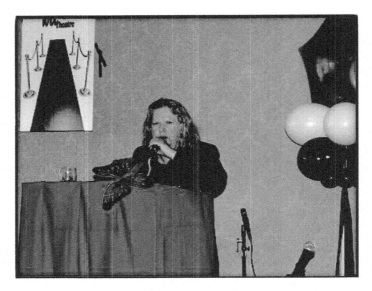

I spent seven years as the emcee of the Red Carpet Awards which was a fun gig. The eighth year I was an awardee for involvement in the theatrical arts.

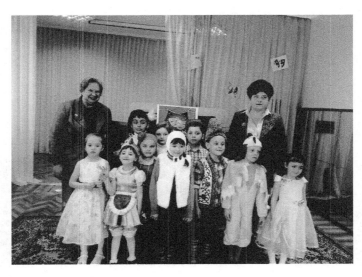

Why did the chicken cross the road? The chicken was going to the theatre. I saw many plays about chickens in Moldova. Happy chickens, angry chickens, crazy chickens. The children are delightful.

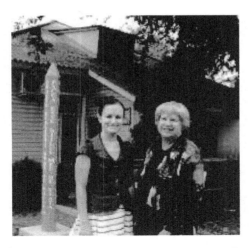

My country partner, Marina Ambrosi and I pose at the peace park in Durlesti, Moldova. Durlesti became the first International City of Peace in a former Soviet Union country. This was a special accomplishment for the community.

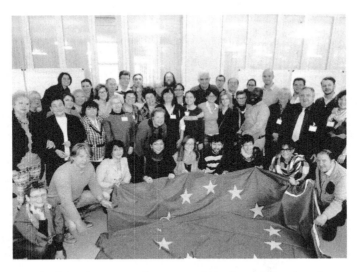

It was wonderful to have travel opportunities for training in other country. This group met in Germany December 2014. Numerous countries were represented. It was productive and interesting. Counting the USA and Moldova my work and personal travels covered 20 countries by the time I returned to America.

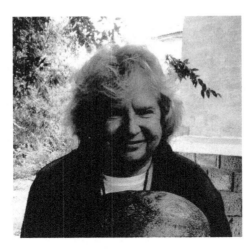

Durlesti my assigned city, celebrated the International Day of Peace and the students presented me with this symbolic loaf of bread September 2014.

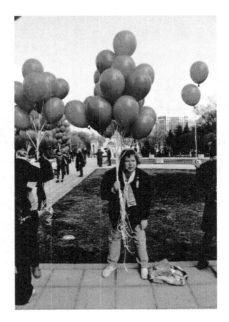

Purple Day brought attention to autism. One of the organizations I worked for helped autistic children. Purple Day in the city center was an annual tradition.

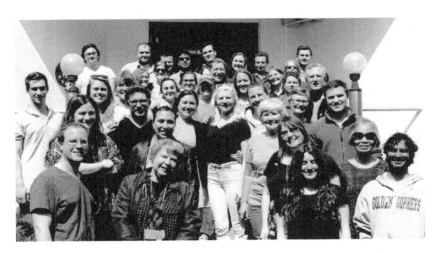

The Peace Corps volunteers pose in front of the Peace Corps headquarters in Moldova. So many talented individuals and fun, too. We worked hard and played hard.

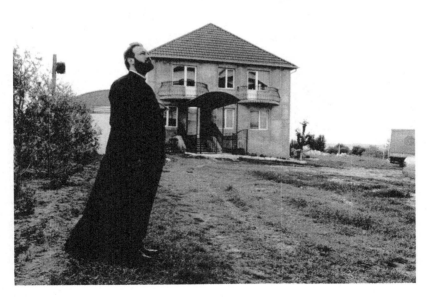

A Moldovan priest standing in the field. A very artsy photo. After the Soviet fall, there were limited clergy. Short term trainings were held to fill the ranks of the ministry to serve the spiritual needs of the people.

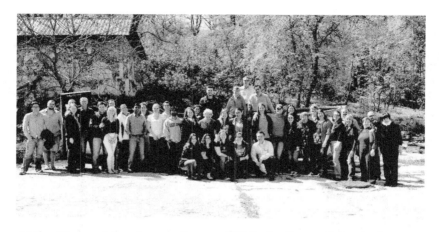

At the Close of Service conference 2015, the Peace Corps volunteers and staff pose in front of an old boat. Soon, everyone would be shipping out sailing to new careers, educational pursuits and new locations.

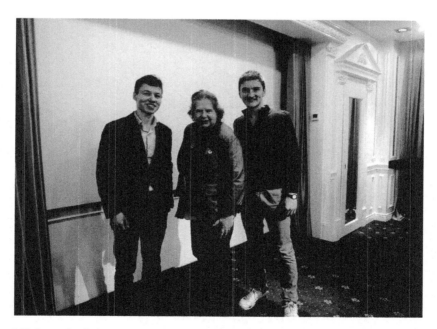

Nick and Liviu two wonderful young men and smart, talented and dedicated as well. We celebrate our third place victory in Diamond Challenge which is a business competition. The boys did a great job.

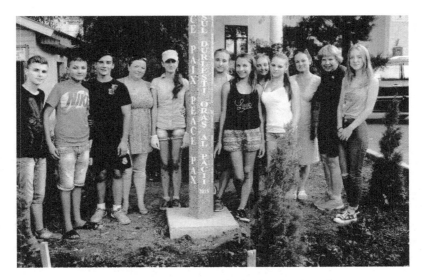

Students surround our new peace pole in Durlesti at the town center. Peace is engraved in several languages all around the pole. The pole became the center of a small park.

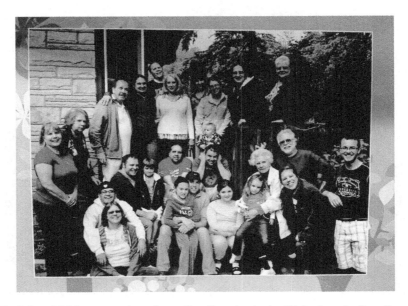

In May 2013, we gather for a family picnic in Ohio just before I go overseas to Peace Corps life.

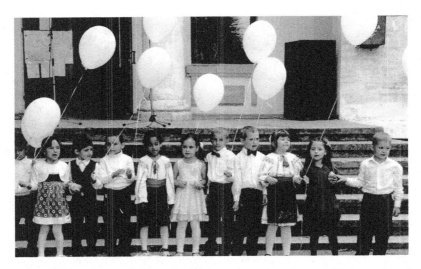

The young students participate in the International Day of Peace. Aren't they adorable? They love to sing and dance.

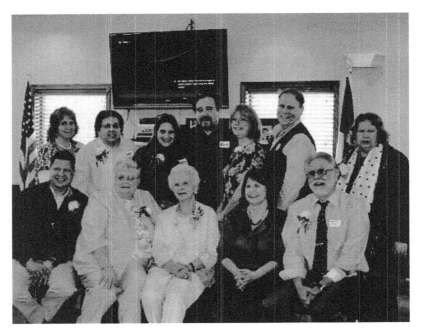

My mother Kathleen and her eleven children celebrating her 90th birthday March 2012.

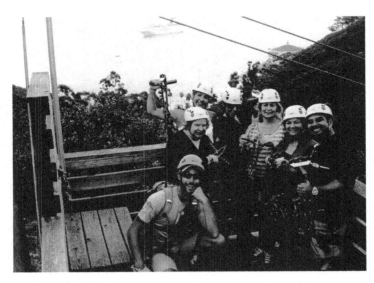

On Catalina Island Oct. 9, 2012 just a few months before leaving for the Peace Corps. It was my birthday and it was most also the birthday of most everyone in this photo. We are going ziplining.

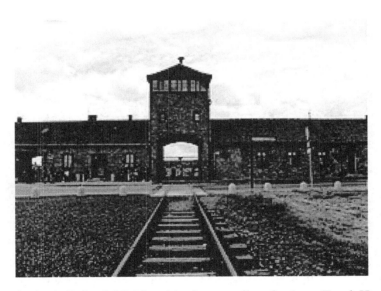

Auschwitz in Poland. Visiting this site as well as the Anne Frank House in the Netherlands were two very touching experiences during my time in Europe. I encourage you to see both.

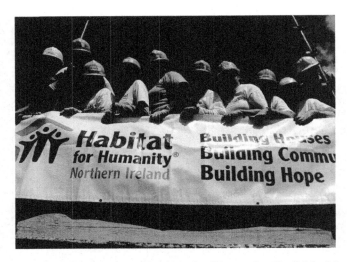

May 2009 participating in a Habitat for Humanity Build in Northern Ireland for a Polish family. I am mostly of Irish and Polish descent so that evens out. This was arranged through St. Monica's my home church in Santa Monica, California.

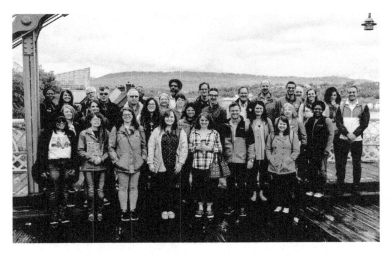

A great opportunity to go on an exploratory tour to Chattanooga, Tennessee with a group from Akron, Ohio sponsored by the Knight Foundation. The tour was informative and generated numerous ideas. This city has done a wonderful job of revitalization with such a lovely energy.

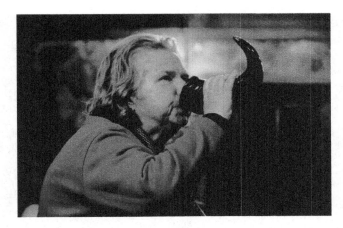

Attending training in Tibilisi, Georgia on the same date as American Thanksgiving. Yes, I chugged it all down. I set it up with fruit juice and that was challenging enough. This was our end of training for a special opportunity I had for the NGO I worked with in Moldova. A great celebration with food, music and dance.

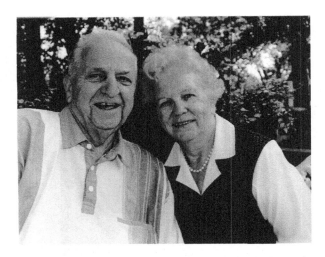

I have a story about Don Grady in this book. This is a photo of my mother and father, Edmund and Kathleen Ostroski. Don Grady's last project before he passed away was a song and video called "The Old Couple". This photo of my parents was featured in that video right before Don and his wife Ginny. So nice. Glad to have connected with Don to make this happen.

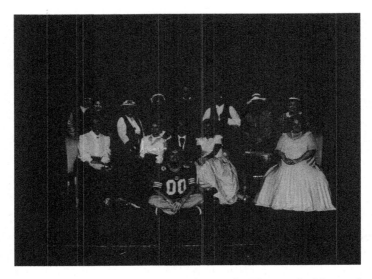

Honored to be cast in this play by the Antic Theatre in November of 2018 in Cuyahoga Falls, Ohio. Such a talented and fun group. The play was about Lizzie Borden and my role was that of a reporter.

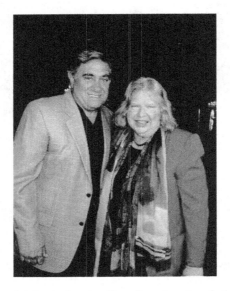

Theatre friend and talented actor Dan Lauria attended the Red Carpet Awards in Los Angeles in 2011 and presented me with my award. It was a great day.

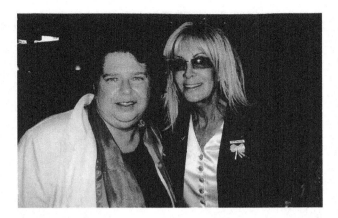

Chatting with actress Joan van Ark during a Red Carpet Award event. Joan was an honoree and later returned twice to present awards and did a lovely introduction of Debbie Reynolds.

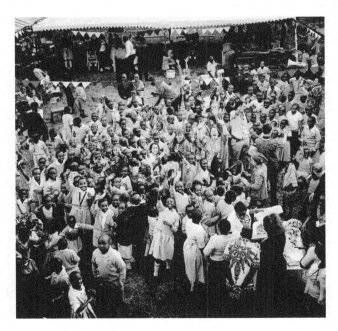

Summer of 2018- a missionary trip to Kenya with a group from St. Monica's Church in Santa Monica, California. This was a great learning experience and very inspiring. What a great group. The Kenyans were wonderful and appreciative of our visit. I loved the children.

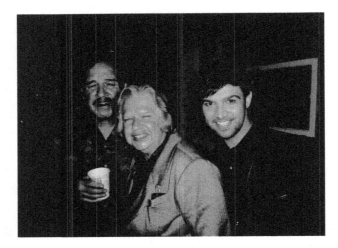

My brother Dennis Ostroski and Chadwick Johnson entertained at my going away to the Peace Corps party in April of 2013 at the Fremont Centre Theatre in South Pasadena. My thanks to Lissa and James Reynolds who run this wonderful theatre for their hospitality in letting us hold the party there. Check out Chandler at www.chandlerjohnson.com

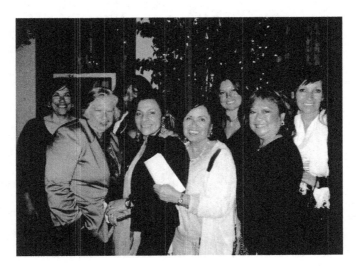

The "angels' from St. Monica. Just a great group of friends in a spiritual sisterhood with a special bond. They came to my farewell party. We shared many social and spiritual moments together including long chats at the ocean at sunset.

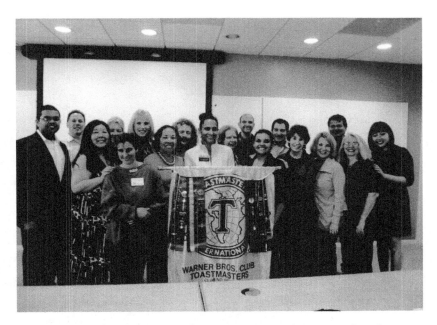

Toastmasters International membership was an important involvement for me in Los Angeles. Going on the lot to attend Warner Brothers Toastmasters was always an interesting adventure and fun.

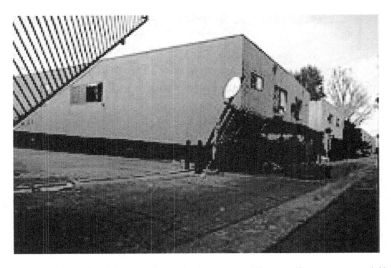

January 1994. The Northridge Earthquake. The walls came tumbling down at my condo and my life changed overnight.

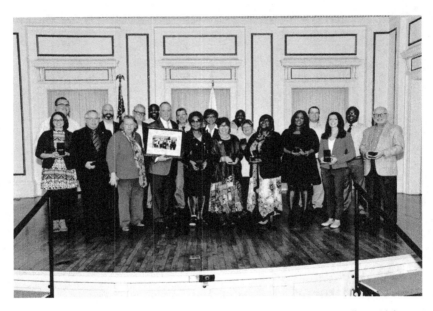

Delighted to be selected for Akron Mayor Dan Horrigan's first Citizens Institute. Wonderful classmates and a great community experience. This photo was taken at our graduation ceremony in 2017.

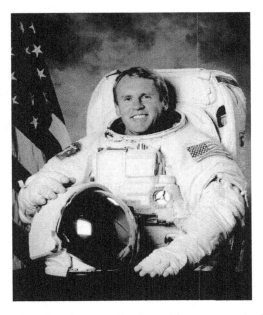

It was fun and educational to spend a day with astronaut Andrew Thomas. He had a great career in space.

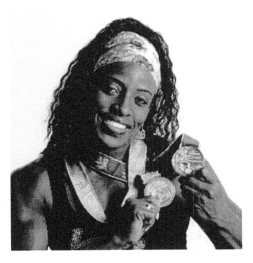

It was fun to spend one day during my Peace Corps service at USA Olympic medalist and WNBA star Ruthie Bolton's basketball camp for young children in Moldova. The kids learned a lot.

Peace and Pieces

Life gives you little bits and pieces. It also gives you lots of people, pets, surprises, and the expected, unexpected, the usual, and the unusual. Each of these is special in its way. Speaking of my favorite pet, our rooster, the next section covers pets, people and other special times and moments.

Section Four

Special Pets, People, Places and Things

Chapter Twenty One

And the Award Goes To

I was very fortunate to receive several awards for my work. These were mostly for writing, directing or creative concepts, but also for public speaking via Toastmasters International speech contests. I was also honored for video editing. I did not perform the technical edits but directed the editor toward certain elements and moods I wanted to create to increase the quality of the productions.

St. Vincent-St. Mary High School in Akron, Ohio honored me in 2011 with the Father Mahar Award for Outstanding Alumni. Several individuals are honored annually. I liked to feel I was recognizing my mother, Kathleen, in receiving this recognition because she was certainly a more outstanding person than I and she was a humble leader. It was delightful that the timing worked out so that the award ceremony was on my mom's birthday. A crowd of more than 300 sang *Happy Birthday* to her. It was an exceptional moment.

The name of the school may be familiar, since it is heard around National Basketball Association circles as the alma mater of NBA player LeBron James. By the way, LeBron is a fellow Mahar Awardee.

I am very conscious that many people are not in positions to receive awards. Being in a creative field such as advertising, opportunities were more present for me, rather than for someone on the cleaning crew or someone who answered the phones. These are all important. Too much is made of awards, and sometimes there are too many problems surrounding them. However, when done right they can serve to inspire, inform and recognize.

Previously, I wrote about the Red Carpet Awards. Sometimes while stumping for nominations, someone would mention they wanted to nominate me. To begin with, I did not feel deserving, compared to the work of so many others, and I said so. But most importantly my job was to seek nominations for others and not for myself. The only reason I was mentioned is that I was there seeking nominations and that made them think of me. I knew, however, that with a little thought they could come up with many others who were even quite more unsung. Finding the unsung was part of the goal of the awards.

Then one day as I was gradually moving toward the Peace Corps and no longer in charge of nominations I was selected. My award was presented to me by a friend, Dan Lauria, who had also been a previous recipient. Dan is probably best known as the father on *The Wonder Years*. He is a great guy and a devoted actor. I was especially honored that I received the 100th Red Carpet Award. That was a goal for the number of awards I wanted to reach as a milestone. It was a nice surprise that this worked out that way and that I was honored to receive it.

The Red Carpet Awards incorporated celebrities, honored poets, acknowledged those who served children and organizations who helped special individuals such as the blind and those with Down Syndrome to be involved in the arts. The arts add so much to our lives. It was touching to acknowledge organizations and individuals who stayed so dedicated to art day in and day out, year by year, decade by decade, lifetime by lifetime. My tagline for the Red Carpet Awards which I discussed in another chapter was "*(The name of the recipient)* -- Please Walk the Red Carpet! This was the time the awardee came to the stage and walked on the red carpet. In this last section of this book, treat yourself as if you are walking on the red carpet of life. You will be in a better position to help others to be honored, bring a community together, and celebrate great things.

"Dwell on the beauty of life. Watch the stars and see yourself running with them."

Marcus Aurelius

Chapter Twenty Two

Sweet Santa's

It is quite common for people to deliver gifts and food to needy families at Christmas time. Sometimes these can be especially touching occasions, and there can be some surprises. There is always a story. Here are just a couple of stories from different parts of the country, and different families, but with the same joy.

Once I was with a group of people delivering holiday gifts to needy families we had signed up to adopt in the San Fernando Valley area of Los Angeles. There was one address we went to, and we just could not find the place. Initially, we thought perhaps we had the wrong address or were not reading the information correctly. We were a bit confused.

Then I went around to what was sort of like a garage but with only a piece of material serving as a door. The cloth was meant to keep out the cold and was even flimsier when it came to providing security. I carefully moved in slightly, drew the curtain aside, and announced myself. We had found our family.

Inside we discovered a mother with a young daughter and a small baby and gently greeted them. I am sure they were somewhat surprised at our sudden appearance and wanted to assure us they were not afraid. We easily overcame the language barrier.

The little girl's eyes sparked with great wonder. I am sure she had probably never seen a wrapped gift in her short life. The dwelling was almost cave-like, with the barest of essentials. I had never seen anything quite like it. It was difficult to even describe it to people. Everything was neat and orderly. It looked as if the family was making the most out of what they had. It was very small. The only "toy" I spotted was the young girl gently holding sort of a basic piece of something that was hard to determine and that was wrapped with a little cloth. It was a sort of doll and a very simple one, but the little item was deeply cherished by that little girl

The child was wide-eyed with wonder to see wrapped gifts and boxes of groceries. I sensed she had never seen anything like this before. There was little in the cupboards, and the small, old, beaten-up refrigerator was essentially bare. There were few clothes or any items at all.

None of us had ever experienced a dwelling so primitive and with so little comforts. It weighed on my mind as we continued our deliveries to other families who had homes, such as a very crowded apartment where many people lived. These seemed more like quite common housing and had a few comforts that are generally expected in apartment living, yet not luxurious by any means.

I had both joy and sadness with this experience. It was a great reminder of how some of our neighbors may be living. The memory of this experience has long stayed with me and had a profound impact on my life.

There are Sweet Santas all over. Another story of delivering gifts to needy families comes to mind. This story is also touching.

A group of church members was delivering presents to needy families in Akron, Ohio. One of the men in the group looked the part and dressed as Santa Claus.

When the group was unloading presents outside an apartment building, a small, shabbily dressed young boy ran out gleefully and grabbed onto Santa's leg. He was holding tightly and was giddy with absolute delight, surprise, and had tears streaming down his slightly dirty cheeks. He shouted, "Mom said you were not going to come this year. But, I knew you would come, Santa. I just knew it!"

The eyes of every member of the group were wet, especially when they realized they were not prepared for a child of this size and age. Still holding tightly to Santa's leg, the boy revealed his family's name and the group sadly discovered his family was not on the list. There were no gifts for them.

Quickly, however, they rounded up what little extra they had and provided those items to the grateful family. Some in the group made a quick assessment of the children; their ages, needs, and sizes and then went out and used their own money to buy more gifts for the family. They pretended that Santa had more presents to be picked up at the North Pole and these would be coming. This allowed them a chance to get some specific gifts for family members.

The young boy delighted in the fact that Santa had made it to his home and would soon be back in record time from the North Pole. He had trust and believed in the magic moment of Santa's arrival. These gentle givers, with their quick and generous actions and follow through, did more than make a family's Christmas special. They inspired hope.

They made a believer out of a child who had little but his firm belief that Santa Claus would find the way. Those Sweet Santas showed up, and thankfully one of them looked just like the real Santa Claus; it made a lasting memory for one little boy and his family.

After all, he had told his mother that Santa would be there, and he believed it. Sure enough, Santa Claus was coming to town. Isn't that what Santa does?

On your life journey, find ways to truly experience those in different life circumstances. Look for ways to be a Sweet Santa even if it is not Christmas and even if you don't believe in Santa. Explore life through the eyes of a child and have that great hope.

"Some are born great, some achieve greatness, and some have greatness thrust upon them."

William Shakespeare

Chapter Twenty Three

Trevor Our Wonder Dog Extraordinaire

Since the beginning of time humanity has been learning and observing from their pets and animals. Pets are an important part of many people's lives.

Everyone needs to have at least one cool pet in their lifetime. (Refrigerators and bathroom roosters probably don't count.)

Trevor was our family dog. Our family of 13 included six girls and five boys from tots through teens, plus a mother and a father.

Trevor came to us as a newborn. He was just a little bundle. Trevor was pretty, noble, and was a mixed breed -- including being part human. He played football with the children in the family and their friends in our large backyard. We played football for fun. Trevor played football and meant business. Trevor could catch touchdown passes with the flair of an NFL star, and he did not like to lose. He jumped, blocked, and tackled with enthusiasm.

Life Lessons from Trevor

- Show enthusiasm
- Learn the skills needed
- Get down to business

- Show a little flair

Trevor played baseball but could not bat. However, he could scoop up ground balls, run the bases with glee and cheer on the team.

- Find your place and do your best
- Overcome your shortcomings
- Cheer everyone on

Trevor sometimes followed the family to school. "Trevor is here" was a frequent shout on the playground. He "guarded' the baby of the family around strangers and relinquished his post when all seemed well. When someone was ill, Trevor stayed at his or her side.

- Take care of your people and be there for them

Trevor made the cover of the local Sunday magazine. A photographer spent the day with Trevor, following him for hours and miles as he met other dogs, took a walk, and more.

- You never know when fame will come. Be ready!
- Let the photographer know what your best side is.

"Look at life from the perspective of your pet. Animals are a wonderful gift from God."

Trish Ostroski

Chapter Twenty Four

Things Can Happen When You Don't Expect It

I had a lot of goals I wrote down at varying periods in my life. It is a great idea to write down something you think might be a bit outrageous and perhaps even impossible

When I moved from Ohio to Los Angeles in 1985, I reviewed many of the goals I had written down. A few were no longer a fit for me or anything I still would like to attain. Things and circumstances change, and we have factors such as age, illness, or other events that may intervene. So, yes, goals should periodically be refined. Technology may even be at play for something that does not exist anymore or at least not in the same manner.

So now back to those outrageous entries in your goals. I wrote down that I would go to the Oscars; this seemed like a sort of pipe dream at the time. However, I did get to go to an Oscar rehearsal where they do the run-through the day before, and you don't even have to dress up. I had a great seat and was in comfy clothing. I spent one Oscar night on the bleachers outside, and later that night Sally Field discovered that we really liked her. I liked sitting on the bleachers and just taking in the whole scene.

I even got to hold an Oscar, which was on display in Hollywood prior to an upcoming ceremony. Yes, it does weigh about nine pounds, and it feels heavy. It would work well as an exercise weight. Surprisingly, it was very much like a media award I had received for writing. It weighed about the same and was in a similar style. So, I was ready for my close-up whether Cecil B. DeMille might ever be looking for me.

I also went to the Ovation Awards, a theatrical awards event, and got to go in the press room and take advantage of that since I was part of the media covering the event. I was fortunate enough to go to many other awards programs and special Hollywood events that included a lot of celebrities and some of the showiest food I had ever seen or tasted.

Once someone offered me 50 free tickets to a Hollywood awards program that was happening in a few days. I tried to dig up as many people as I could in only a short bit of time. This event was beyond my expectations and included a lovely meal before the program. While I was waiting for some of the others, Mickey Rooney dined alone at an adjacent table. It was nice to get the tickets and to take other people along.

Due to my involvement with one of the arts high schools in Los Angeles, I received an invitation to one of their special events. I was expecting a seat in the nosebleed section, but to my surprise, my guest and I were seated in the first row. We could pretty much reach out and touch Josh Groban, Bob Newhart, Barry Manilow, and several others who performed that great night.

If you put this all together, it pretty much equals going to the Oscars without being treated like cattle, which is often the case even for nominees who are nominated in "lesser" categories or for those who are not names or celebrities.

Be sure to add some outrageous ideas to your goals. Things can appear piece by piece if not all at once. Sometimes coming close may be enough. Enjoy!

"I think one's feelings waste themselves in words; they ought all be distilled into actions which bring result."

Florence Nightingale

Chapter Twenty Five

At Seventeen

One Los Angeles night I was driving from Santa Monica to the San Fernando Valley on surface streets. I was driving through the night and just thinking. Janis Ian's epic song *At Seventeen* came on the radio. I had heard this song many times and truly loved the poetry and the deep meaning of each phrase. As she delicately sang each line I was amazed at the insightful poetry that most everyone could relate to, even if often not expressed.

I thought that I would love to hear the thoughts behind each line and what the writer was feeling. These little whimsical requests are a great way to keep alert while on a long drive in the dark Los Angeles night. But never did I think my request would be granted.

I submitted a short play I wrote, *For Better... For Worse,* to a women's art festival sponsored by the Los Angeles Women's Theatre Project. My play was selected for a staging. The festival was to be in Palm Springs, and Janis Ian was to be a special guest artist. Janis performed a concert; it was a great experience to sit there and listen to her lovely voice and hear the variety of songs she performed

The big plus was that there would be a sort of class and discussion with Janis in an intimate setting with just a couple dozen people. I was one of them. To my delight, she began to go through *At Seventeen* line by line, thought by thought, flow by flow. I was truly mesmerized and flabbergasted that my request to have that song analyzed line by line was granted that day. The piece is a superb application of the poetic process that creates a song, tells a story, delivers a message, and gives you something to think about. Today few of the songs being written do that. I admired the creative and careful thought Ms. Ian put to each and every word and phrase.

Before Janis began her review of the song, she talked about other things and directed a couple of questions to me, apparently recognizing by my body language and responses that I was a bit more a writer than a performer, although I did both.

Remember, someone must write the script, poem, prose or whatever, for it to be recited or delivered to an audience. I was truly light-headed and in awe as I left the session. I also had lots of inspiration stirring within.

It was a thrill to see the play I wrote and directed on stage at the festival. It was a bigger thrill to have that time with Janis Ian. It was an even bigger thrill that my wish on that late-night drive in Los Angeles had come true. Yes, sometimes someone is out there listening to you. So, my advice is to put things out there, soak up the special moments, and tune into the poetry of life.

"In special moments of thought, great insight can arrive. Sometimes it enters subtly, and other times it arrives all gift wrapped. No matter the way it enters, it is a great gift."

Trish Ostroski

Bonus---The Complete Lyrics to At Seventeen

At Seventeen
Janis Ian

I learned the truth at seventeen
That love was meant for beauty queens
And high school girls with clear skinned smiles
Who married young and then retired
The valentines I never knew
The Friday night charades of youth
Were spent on one more beautiful
At seventeen I learned the truth
And those of us with ravaged faces
Lacking in the social graces
Desperately remained at home
Inventing lovers on the phone
Who called to say "Come dance with me"
And murmured vague obscenities
It isn't all it seems
At seventeen
A brown eyed girl in hand-me-downs
Whose name I never could pronounce
Said, "Pity, please, the ones who serve
They only get what they deserve"
And the rich relationed hometown queen
Marries into what she needs
With a guarantee of company
And haven for the elderly
Remember those who win the game
Lose the love they sought to gain
In debentures of quality
And dubious integrity
Their small-town eyes will gape at you
In dull surprise when payment due

THERE'S A ROOSTER IN MY BATHROOM

Exceeds accounts received
At seventeen
To those of us who knew the pain
Of valentines that never came
And those whose names were never called
When choosing sides for basketball
It was long ago and far away
The world was younger than today
When dreams were all they gave for free
To ugly duckling girls like me
We all play the game, and when we dare
To cheat ourselves at solitaire
Inventing lovers on the phone
Repenting other lives unknown
They call and say, "Come dance with me"
And murmur vague obscenities
At ugly girls like me
At seventeen

Songwriters: Janis Ian

Chapter Twenty Six

See You Sooner

While reading the book *Home Before Morning: The Story of an Army Nurse in Vietnam* by Lynda Van Devanter, I was deeply touched by the inside story of Vietnam as told from a women's point of view -- and an army nurse at that.

Lynda Van Devanter was a girl-next-door type who was a bubbly cheerleader and went to Catholic schools. She enjoyed sports and her large family, which included four sisters and her parents. After high school, she attended nursing school and in 1969 joined the U.S. Army as a nurse.

She shipped off to Vietnam full of idealistic views. However, that idealism soon vanished as she saw friends die and was burdened by long and arduous work hours. She dealt not only with the long hours but also the cramped, ill-equipped, understaffed operating rooms. Each day she found the very foundations of her thinking continually challenged as she moved more in touch to what war and the situation really was.

This book had a profound effect on me. One interesting sidelight was that I wanted to share this book with my friend Lori Brenner Balsley, who was in nurse's training. When I saw her about a week after finishing the book, I discovered she had also been reading the book at the same time I was. It was one of those books you could not put down.

Upon further research and reflection, I discovered Sharon Lane. Sharon grew up not far from me just south of Canton, Ohio. Interestingly, my friend Lori had the same alma mater as Sharon. They both attended Canton South High School.

Sharon Lane ended up joining the Army and serving as a nurse in Vietnam. After being in the country for just a few weeks, she was assigned the night schedule . Just minutes from completing her shift, Sharon was killed by enemy fire. Eight women died in military service in Vietnam. Sharon was the only one of the eight who died from enemy fire. There are 58,317 names on the Vietnam Wall. Eight are women. Sharon Lane is one of them.

It is a profound experience to see the Vietnam Wall. I encourage you to go to Washington, D.C. to see it. If you cannot go there, sometimes there are touring Vietnam Walls that may be set up in your community. Take some time to experience it.

People leave little gifts and notes along the Wall. Some trace the names of loved ones on to pieces of paper. Observing all of this and seeing familiar names is an emotional experience.

You might benefit from some additional information about Sharon Lane. Just four days before being mortally wounded by enemy fire while working in the 312th Evacuation Hospital in Chu Lai, Republic of Vietnam, First Lieutenant Sharon Ann Lane signed a letter to her parents in her characteristically upbeat manner, *See You Sooner.*

Writing to her parents about the heat, those in her care, and the movie she missed the night before, Lane assured her parents that things were quiet at her station. Ironically, within days of writing that letter, Sharon was killed.

I was inspired to write a play about Sharon Lane, told as a series of letters I imagined as correspondence between herself and her parents and also between Sharon and a high-school friend character that I made up. I entitled the play. *See You Sooner.* It was performed as a staged reading at the Stella Adler Theatre on Hollywood Blvd. in the heart of Hollywood. Stella Adler was a legendary actress and acting teacher.

The day my play was being staged, I had a memorable view of Hollywood Blvd. from an upper floor just before going on stage. It was a special moment to bring this story alive. Two childhood friends, Jim and Sallie Carroll, were in attendance as was my brother Dennis. Dennis provided good feedback on audience reaction. It was a thrill to have this staged and share the story of a brave woman. Legendary actress Bette Rae was perfect as Sharon's mother. She passed away later, while I was on my way to join my fellow Peace Corps volunteers in Philadelphia.

More about Sharon Lane. Her nursing assignment was physically and emotionally challenging, yet she declined transfers to other assignments. She spent her off-duty time taking care of the most critically injured American soldiers in the surgical ICU.

She thrived despite the demanding schedule and was adored and respected by co-workers and patients alike.

In the early morning of June 8, 1969, the 312th Evacuation Hospital was struck by rockets fired by the Viet Cong. Two were killed, and 27 were wounded. Sharon Lane was killed instantly.

For her service in Vietnam, Sharon Ann Lane was awarded the Purple Heart, the Bronze Star with "V" device, the National Defense Service Medal, the Vietnam Service Medal, the National Order of Vietnam Medal, and the Vietnamese Gallantry Cross.

She received further recognition from individuals and organizations who honored Lane in a variety of ways by naming sections of hospitals after her; in 1969 the Daughters of the American Revolution named her Outstanding Nurse of the year. The Canton, Ohio Chapter of the Vietnam Veterans of America officially changed its name to the Sharon Lane Chapter #199. Streets in Denver, Colorado and Fort Belvoir, Virginia have been named in her honor. Even after all these years, Sharon Lane remains an important symbol representing the sacrifices and service of the thousands of American women who served in the Vietnam War.

A lot of years passed between my reading *Home Before Morning* and writing a short play about Army nurse Sharon Lane. This demonstrates that thoughts and ideas come to you and you need to serve them to bring them to life in some manner even if it takes time. This book is another example of that.

When a story, an individual, or some entity inspires you, be sure to share it with others. After all, everyone needs inspiration. Emulate the dedication, devotion, and caring demonstrated by people like Sharon Lane instead of wasting time hearing about some of the silly escapades of celebrities.

"Truth is powerful, and it prevails."

Sojourner Truth

Bonus----The Play --*See You Sooner*
(Note as a special gift to readers,
I have included *See You Sooner* for your reading enjoyment.)

See You Sooner
By Trish Ostroski

(Narrator)

Sharon A. Lane was born July 7, 1943, in Zanesville, Ohio. She later moved with her family to a rural area near Canton, Ohio. After graduating from high school, she attended Aultman Nursing School and then began a nursing career followed by a short stint in the business world. Sharon heard her country calling and joined the U.S. Army Nurse Corps in 1968. Little did she know that this would be the start of something that would eventually put her down in history.

She began her basic training in Texas with the rank of Second Lieutenant and was assigned to Denver, Colorado where she worked in the tuberculosis and cardiac wards. She received a promotion to First Lieutenant, and after a brief stop at Travis Air Force Base in California, she was soon on her way to Vietnam in April 1969.

She arrived at the 312th Evac Hospital at Chu Lai and went to work in the Intensive Care ward and was later assigned to the Vietnamese

Ward. She worked six days a week, 12 hours per day, in this ward or intensive care.

During the early morning hours of June 8, 1969, a Soviet-built 122-mm rocket slammed into ward 4 of the 312th Evacuation Hospital in Chu Lai, Vietnam. The 24 year old Lt. Sharon A. Lane died instantly. Though seven other American military nurses lost their lives serving in Vietnam, Lt. Lane was the only American servicewoman killed as a direct result of enemy fire throughout the war.

Sharon was often noted for using the phrase..."see you sooner" as opposed to the popularized..."see you later". This piece is composed as a series of letters as imagined by the playwright that Sharon writes to her family and to her friends conveying thoughts she may have been thinking in regards to her experiences.

The last letter is from Sharon's mother to her deceased daughter.

(Staging—actor on stool, reads the letter to the audience—dressed in military fatigue top)

April 17, 1969

Dear Mom and Dad,

I am excited about serving in Vietnam. I look forward to putting my nursing skills to good use and serving humanity. When I briefly switched to business while putting my nursing career on hold—it was because I felt I was not being fulfilled as a nurse.

In the military, here stateside, and soon in Vietnam I know I will be both challenged and rewarded. I am certain I will be serving my fellow human beings.

I know you are concerned about my assignment in Vietnam. But please don't be. Hey -- nurses don't die in Vietnam unless it is from long hours of work with so much to do—ha- ha. And you know what dad always says—'hard work never killed anyone"—so I should be plenty safe. And you know my philosophy---

I am thankful for this day. I am thankful for good health.

Today I will go through the day inwardly relaxed and outwardly alert.

I will pay more attention to the things outside of me and less attention

to the things inside me. I will enjoy my food, the weather, my work, and the people around me. I believe I will be given the strength

to meet whatever problems come to me. I will do my tasks one at a time,

and not try to cross all my bridges at once. All my love—See you sooner,

Sharon

(Actor takes on a youthful tone)

May 5, 1969

Dear Linda,

Thank you for your recent letter. It is hard to believe that you guys are already starting work on our ten year high school class reunion. Gee- that it is only two years away. Time flies. Well, when you decide the date and all—please let me know—I will put it in my datebook—ha-ha. I will be out of Vietnam by then—but perhaps not out of the military. Who knows where I will be and what adventure I might be up to?

I work 12 hour days—six days a week. Life is no picnic -but I see the value of the work I do—every day—in the faces of the young guys I care for.

It is hard to believe that a few of the guys in our class have been killed in Vietnam. I still picture Bobby Jordan dancing at the record hops and cruising around in that old car of his. Hard to imagine—he was so full of life and had so many hopes. I went to the sophomore homecoming dance with Ted Dexter. Even then he had plans to join the military right after graduation. He was so looking forward to a career in the military like his dad. Ted had such bravado about him. He seemed so invincible, and now he is gone. One second you are there…and then you are not.

There are a lot of guys like Bobby and Ted here in Vietnam. So young, so sure.

You asked about guys? Ha-ha. I do meet a lot of single guys. Well, I guess you mean romance and love. In my few short weeks here— well nothing like that—But wait—yes there is a lot of love, and that is what gets me through the days and the nights.

Just yesterday I was taking care of a critically injured soldier who had little chance from the get go—even though we encouraged his spirits. He looked at me--- and said—"Sharon I never even really had a girlfriend." I held his hand tightly, and he embraced mine.

In the wee hours, he slipped through the bond from earth to heaven. He looked so young—yet in some ways so old. I found his prom photo in his wallet posing shyly with a young girl who looked as shy and innocent as he did. Hard to believe that photo was only a year old. He was just a year out of high school—and had not even reached his 19th birthday. He had not even had a real girlfriend. That was something he was looking forward to. He was holding my hand when he passed away. You might say Linda—I have experienced love—on a level as never before. And that is what gets me through the days and through the nights.

We have a motto—

On my watch, you will never be alone. I will hold your hand and wipe the tears in this land so far away from home.

When you see guys with body parts missing and suffering badly you hurt. You see guys feeling alone, and you feel alone as well. I see guys differently than I ever have before. It is not about who has a cool car, a cute haircut, or is even a great dancer. Stuff like that seems so unimportant now. After a few days here—life looks a lot different. I have seen guys as human beings as never before. Being in Vietnam is like being in another world. You couldn't believe that it was real, that you weren't just on another planet

Ah--romantic love will come—but I just think that is down the line right now. I have more important things now.

Hey girl—say hello to the gang.

Be sure to write,

See you sooner,

Love --Sharon

May 30, 1969

Dear Mom and Dad,

I will soon be assigned to the night shift. No worries about getting up early in the morning—after my extensive social life-- ha-ha. The shifts are long and intensive—but in many ways, the time flies by, and you hate to leave because there is so much to do. But you know of course that you need your rest as well.

That one day off a week—comes as a just reward to get some extra sleep, write letters do laundry and maybe even have some time to write in my journal or read a book while listening to some music.

Sure pleasures are few—but it is such a pleasure to be a nurse and serve proudly.

I have seen more and learned more in a few weeks than I probably would have learned in 10 years in stateside nursing.

It is never boring, and one is constantly asking what more might one do. It just seems like it is never enough. So many patients. So many needs. So little time. So very little time.

One of the 'rules' is that nurses are not allowed to cry. The wounded and dying men in our care need our strength; we cannot indulge in the luxury of our own feelings. That day off —once a week—is a good time to shed a few tears in privacy with your thoughts. I sometimes cry myself to sleep-but no one sees that but me.

If you talk to Linda—tell her I will write soon.

And as for you guys and the family—See you sooner,

All my love,

Sharon

(Actor takes on reflective tone)

June 8, 1969

Dear Journal,

The night is both quiet and yet busy. My shift will be ending in less than an hour. I am just wrapping up some final details and preparing for my relief. I will be home before morning as we nurses say---meaning I will be leaving right around 6 am when Judy Daniels my relief reports in.

I hear some noise in the distance—but yet—it is quiet —even though there is that constant background noise. But that is how Vietnam is—both quiet and full of noise at the same time. So quiet —so loud. So full of peace---so full of war. So full of bravery— and yet we shrink within. That is what days are like in Vietnam. That is what nights are like in Vietnam—just that darker part of the day when you hope to see the dawn in more ways than one. After a few days- I am getting used to the night shift. Gee—this is my 40th day in Vietnam. Forty days and Forty nights—gee—like Christ in the dessert- --like Lent. Forty days----forty nights. So short and yet so long. What a change forty days can bring.

It is 5:30 am —I will be leaving very soon. Yes, leaving very soon. My work is nearly done. (A brief pause)

(Performer wraps self in the American flag)

5: 50 am---

Shots ring out. I am hit—a bullet seeps in me—you have that revelation, and the pain is intense—but it happens so fast---I am on the floor—I hover between—earth and heaven—I am seeing my body bleeding below. I want to pull back to earth—and yet something pulls me to what is beyond—my life flashes in front of me---it is like an instant—it is like an eternity. They say I died instantly—is anything really that instant?

Bleeding to death—it goes so fast--but you have those moments of realization--so fleeting. I am a nurse. Nurses don't cry. Nurses don't die. This cannot be happening. It must be a dream. It must be a nightmare. Nurses don't die in Vietnam. Nurses don't get killed in Vietnam. Nurses don't get killed by bullets in Vietnam. How can they? I am here to heal—but I cannot heal myself.

(Pause)

The news of the action reaches the evening news in Ohio. While both of my parents are watching —a military vehicle pulls up to my parents' house. Mom wastes no punches and no steps and even before my dad gets to the door—my mom asks —"Is she dead"?—and hears the affirmative.

(Pause)

Oh, journal—you have let me share my thoughts—you have been my paper friend here in Vietnam—and always at the ready. You were there for me to share my thoughts when bullets rang in the distance. You were there for me to share my thoughts when guys died in my arms. You were there for me to share my thoughts when I thought I could not think anymore. You let me share thoughts that sometimes were difficult to write and thoughts that were even more difficult to comprehend.

But this is my last entry, and it came sooner than I thought. All of life came sooner—sooner than I thought.

(Fade)

(Women sits in a rocker wearing shawl—takes on a motherly/elderly tone— —performer is writing a letter)

March 30, 2009

Dear Sharon,

It is Woman's History Month here now. And I was thinking of you and your place in history---of course as your mother I think of you every day as a mother remembers a daughter who died too soon. It is amazing the history you have created. I miss you, and I miss your dad—hard to believe it has been almost 30 years since he passed away. Lucky him--He got to see you sooner. Your brother and sister are nearby, and all of your nieces and nephews continue to make us all proud. You would have loved every one of them. I wish you could have known them. I wish they could have known you.

Your place in history is very special—although I always say—Sharon would not have wanted all of this—she was just a regular girl—just our Sharon—just a regular girl—but oh so special. You were a wonderful daughter who was gone much too soon.

The Daughters of the American Revolution named you 'Outstanding Nurse of the Year' in 1969, and honored you with 'The Anita Newcomb McGee Medal.' The Fitzsimons Hospital where you served in Denver named its recovery room the 'Lane Recovery Suite.' Several of the schools that you have attended honored you in many ways. Aultman Hospital opened the Sharon Lane Women's Center. There are two roads named for you at your former army assignments, and there is a Sharon Lane Volunteer Center in Texas. There is a permanent display in your honor at the Ohio Society of Military History in Massillon, Ohio.

There is more. The Sharon Ann Lane Foundation is building a clinic at Chu Lai Vietnam where you served. The Foundation envisions this Clinic as a Bridge of

Friendship between two former enemies. The hope is to provide returning Vietnam Veterans, visiting Americans, Vietnamese and all who enter healing, and understanding —so even from the beyond as you did on earth—you are still providing healing and understanding—and friendship ----the true mission of the army nurse. You provided a bridge of friendship to people from both worlds.

This March has been a tough one here in Ohio—a bit too wintry for me. But being inside has given me lots of time to think—and think about you. Oh how I miss you. Oh how I miss the times we would have spent together. And you know what—I am nearly 90—the aches and pains are more frequent. The days are a little harder and the nights a little more lonely. And my dear Sharon—I know now---I will see you sooner---sooner than you think. (Fade Out)

END

Notes—thanks to Bette Rae who has now moved to heaven and Mary Burkin for their participation in this production. Also, to the Los Angeles Women's Theatre Project and the Stella Adler Theatre in Hollywood. Thank you for the opportunity.

Chapter Twenty Seven

Things that Just Pop Up — But Lead to Good

I was away at a weekend workshop shared with fellow employees who also worked at Precision Dynamics Corporation. I checked my voicemail at work from the hotel. I had a message from a local nun. If you went to Catholic schools, you sometimes might think to yourself, well now, what does this little nun want from me now?

But sometimes you can get a cool request. The request was for me to be a photographer for actor Richard Dreyfuss at an awards banquet. Mr. Dreyfuss was being honored by Valley Family Center, a local service agency in San Fernando, California. This was shortly before the movie *Mr. Holland's Opus* came out. Publicity about this upcoming movie had appeared, however, and many teachers attended the program due to this interest. *Mr. Holland's Opus* was about a music teacher who had a strong desire to write a symphony while balancing that with the needs of his family and his teaching career.

I had a fun night interacting with Mr. Dreyfuss and members of his family, as well as many other attendees. During all the activity, I forced myself to be reminded that on occasion a nun might just have a fun assignment for you. I had often taken snapshots and photos at other events, so it was nice to add one more opportunity like this to my list.

Which reminds me, I even went to jail with a celebrity, all in good fun for a fundraiser. Former professional football player turned actor Fred Dryer had played a police detective in the long-running series *Hunter*. The series became famous for the line, "Works for me." There was a local fundraiser where people get arrested for silly charges, and you pay to get them out of jail. I followed along with a video camera to record Detective Hunter arresting "hardened" criminals in the name of charity. It was a fun day, and *it worked for me*. Always take the phone calls you receive from nuns unless you are pretty sure they are carrying a ruler.

"There is no charm equal to tenderness of heart."

Jane Austen

Chapter Twenty Eight

A Day with an Astronaut — Flying High

I was tasked by my employer to locate a guest speaker for a program to be held for the company's annual sales meeting. I discovered that NASA (National Aeronautics and Space Administration) had a program that would lend astronauts -- with rules and procedures -- to allow them to do presentations to the public. I thought this to be great public relations jewel, so pursued it.

Initially, my request did not garner any results. Keep in mind the astronauts must balance these requests with workloads. They were expected to fulfill a certain number of speaking requests each year, however.

I had booked another speaker, and then one day I got a phone call from a gentleman with a lovely Australian accent. This was my first introduction to Andrew Thomas. Here is a little more about him from his NASA biography. He had not gone into space at the time of my phone call. However, he would total 177 days in space, including serving aboard the Russian Space Station Mir for 130 days.

Dr. Andrew Thomas was selected by NASA in March 1992 and reported to the Johnson Space Center in August 1992. In August 1993, following a year of training, he was appointed a member of the astronaut corps and was qualified for assignment as a mission specialist on space shuttle flight crews.

While awaiting assignment, Dr. Thomas supported shuttle launch and landing operations as an Astronaut Support Person (ASP) at the Kennedy Space Center. He also provided technical support to the Space Shuttle Main Engine project, the Solid Rocket Motor project and the External Tank project at the Marshall Space Flight Center in Huntsville, Alabama. In June 1995, Dr. Thomas was named as payload commander for STS-77 and flew his first flight in space on Endeavour in May 1996. He next trained at the Gagarin Cosmonaut Training Center in Star City, Russia, in preparation for a long-duration flight. In 1998, he served as Board Engineer 2 aboard the Russian Space Station Mir for 130 days. From August 2001 to November 2003, Dr. Thomas served as Deputy Chief of the Astronaut Office. Dr. Thomas completed his fourth space flight on STS-114 and retired from NASA in February 2014.

Since we had already booked another speaker, I suggested ways that the program would benefit from both speakers and be exciting for other workers not aligned with the sales meeting. They would have an opportunity to see and meet an astronaut. With a little persuasion on my part, the proposal was approved.

I picked up Andy at the Burbank Airport on his arrival. A strapping and handsome blond approached the sign I had with his name on it. His Australian charm, wit, and intelligence quickly came forth. He was very polite and had great insight and respect for others. I picked him up at his hotel the next day, and we drove together to the sales meeting.

Andy spoke at the sales meeting, toured the factory and was such a polished public relations vehicle with his wit, communications, and stories. It was a delight to meet and know him. After his visit, we exchanged the occasional card or letter. It was a thrill to follow his adventures when he was in space for lengthy durations.

Thinking back about picking him up in my Ford Escort and driving the Los Angeles streets at about thirty miles an hour when we were moving and not in one of LA's famous traffic jams, I reflected what a difference in speed that street driving and the astronaut journey Andy Thomas took. We have fast journeys and those that are slow in life. They all serve their purpose. Keep exploring and continue to seek new information. Try to fly high now and then. Who knows? You may even fly high with an astronaut.

"To have courage for whatever comes in life -- everything lies in that."

St. Teresa of Avila

Chapter Twenty Nine

When You Add Nebraska to Fahrenheit 451, What Do You Get?

You get a chance to connect two wonderful and talented people.

As a theatrical critic, I reviewed plays and musical shows in more than 100 venues in and around Los Angeles. One of my favorite places was the Fremont Centre Theatre in South Pasadena. Lissa and James Reynolds manage the theatre. You may know James as a longtime actor on *Days of Our Lives*. Lissa also appeared on the show and both have a long list of stage credits.

I just love the vibe of this particular theatre and its hospitality. In fact, I so loved this place that I had my going-away party there when I was leaving for the Peace Corps. Such a wonderful night.

My theatrical work took me to the Fremont to review the play *Fahrenheit 451*. This play was the adaptation of the book of the same name by author Ray Bradbury published in 1953 and is regarded as one of his best works. The novel presents a future American society where books are outlawed, and "firemen" burn any that are found. *Fahrenheit 451* is the presumed temperature at which a book can catch fire, and that is why this title was used.

I would be reviewing the play adapted from the book, and as a nice surprise, the theatre had seated me next to Mr. Bradbury. I had asked actress Angela McEwen to be my guest and to surprise her; I offered her the seat next to Ray Bradbury. I discovered that Angela had taken a class from him and they had not seen each other in years. So this worked out better than I expected for both individuals.

Just before my leaving for the Peace Corps, Angela took me out for lunch and had a wonderful story of how director Alexander Payne met her at her house to talk to her and cast her in the film *Nebraska,* starring Bruce Dern. Angela was so excited in relating the details and *Nebraska* gained much acclaim. I was so happy for her. Angela starred as Bruce Dern's former girlfriend and had a shining moment. This was well deserved for an actress who delayed her career while raising her children and is truly one of the sweetest people I have ever met.

While overseas, I got an occasional email from Angela saying she was ill and was having some medical issues. I never got an opportunity to see *Nebraska* while in Europe. But on December 20, 2015, I received a special holiday opportunity to watch a free movie on my computer. I quickly chose *Nebraska* and enjoyed it, especially Angela's engaging performance. After watching the movie, I sent Angela a short email praising her performance and sharing my enjoyment of the movie. The next day I found out that she had passed away shortly after I watched her movie. I was happy to get that opportunity, just as she was moving to heaven.

Ray Bradbury passed away in 2012. I was grateful for having the opportunity to reconnect Angela and Ray and thankful for their contributions to the arts. In a way I got a front-row seat to observe all of that.

Please note that connections can often be very powerful. Surprise people when you can.

"Happiness is the only good. The time to be happy is now. The place to be happy is here. The way to be happy is to make others so."

Robert Green Ingersoll

Section Five

And One More Thing

Chapter Thirty

Followership

(I wrote this article for my high school newspaper when I was 16. Have not changed it. In some ways I may have been ahead of the times.)

Followership! What's That?

Followership? Ever hear of it? Ever wonder about it?

Webster has omitted the word from the dictionary, but just because it isn't in the dictionary doesn't mean it does not mean it doesn't exist.

Followership is important and is becoming more important all the time.

Daily life is so varied that we can follow in many ways but lead in only a few fields.

The word followership implies "follow through" getting the job done. Followers don't receive much praise or publicity for the jobs they do, but they rate tops in humility.

Hard work is put into all school activities. The chairmen or presidents can't do the job alone. They need good workers. These are the followers who may not be the head of any one thing but are workers for many things.

Leadership is being stressed today more than ever. Books are written about it, people talk about it, and students are rated on it.

However, the real leaders don't always march at the head of a parade. "Take charge guys" are often at a premium, but every group can use "just another follower."

Updates

When I wrote this piece in the 1960s, the word "followership" was not in the dictionary, but it is now. As a teenager, I felt I was coining a phrase. To me, I was using a word I never heard before. Chances are it was out there, but had not been placed in the dictionary. Followership is defined as the capacity or willingness to follow a leader. There have been thousands of books written about leadership and only a handful of books published about followership. The numbers for both topics continue to rise.

I mention this topic because I see that I was on to something when I was just a teen, and it was fun to take a look at that article. (Try this for fun. Go back and read something you wrote as a youth. What might your younger self teach you? How did you look at the world.?)

Here is what I would like to share as an adult. Leadership is important and who, and what we follow is also important. There are only two things that can change your life and therefore inspire change in the world around you.

Either something new comes into your life, or something new comes from within you. Those events inspire change. The important thing is to never let your circumstances or your past limit your visions for the future. Don't limit the vision for others. What you follow and who you choose to follow will define your life.

Just one more thing. We have all heard of common sense. However, this does not mean that common sense is a common practice. We can often get caught up in what we are leading and following and not have the best sense about it. Looking back to myself as a teenager, I think these were the underlying points I was striving to stress. We know leadership can be good and it can be bad. The same principle applies to the lesser reviewed act of followership.

Leadership is not just done by the leader, and followership is not just done by followers. If leaders are to be credited with setting a vision for an organization and inspiring followers to action, then followers should receive credit for the work required to make the vision a reality.

"Wise men speak because they have something to say; Fools because they have to say something."

Plato

Chapter Thirty One

All Good Stuff

I have attended numerous seminars and conferences. I am going to share advice that continually presented and expanded upon during many of these sessions. These will just be brief and possibly serve as a reminder of something you already know. There are plenty of books and resources for you to dig deeper on these topics.

Daily Meditation

Meditation is something everyone can do to improve their mental and emotional health. You can do it anywhere, and you don't need any special equipment, and there are many resources including groups and online help.

There are a variety of styles of meditation to use depending on your personal goals and your style. You only need a few minutes a day and those few minutes can make a big difference.

Meditation can reduce stress, control anxiety, promote emotional health, enhance self-awareness, and lengthen attention span. Also, it may reduce age-related memory loss, improve sleep, help control pain, lowers blood pressure and many meditators feel the practice generates feelings of kindness.

Daily Prayer

Prayer is something that can be worked in while you are driving or doing something else. You can also have a dedicated prayer time. The start and end of the day may be a perfect time for you to pray.

Here are some tips: Keep it simple, pray often, open your heart, use your own words or choose a standard prayer to use as a template. Lastly, listen expectantly for a response.

You can sit, stand, or kneel and you could even stand on your head. Your hands can be open or closed, and your eyes can be open or closed. You can pray anywhere such as in a church, at home, or outside; in the morning or at night just depending on personal preferences.

Gratitude

Keep a gratitude journal or make a daily list of five things for which you are thankful. You may be surprised at things you take for granted. It may be interesting to note all the varied aspects of life that you can offer joyful gratitude for experiencing so much.

Journal

Review your day and reflect for the next day. Would you handle something different next time? Are there lessons for the day? Do you have any new insight or see something differently? The process of journaling compels us to access our memories of an experience and then creates another more recent memory of that experience.

By journaling, you create a physical record of those memories that you can reference in the future. Many people who look back on their journals appreciate their experiences with "ordinary" days rather than days when something unusual may have occurred.

Writing by hand as compared to typing on a computer can add some benefits to your journaling. Handwriting is becoming a thing of the past to many people. However, note that handwriting increases learning comprehension, engages and stimulates your brain, slows down mental aging and unleashes creativity. The process of writing by hand has been known to decrease depression and anxiety, enhances focus, and can combat dyslexia. Write On!

Breaks, Breathing, and Exercise

Your day will be more productive if you take breaks and work in some exercise. Do some occasional stretching, take a short walk, concentrate on your breathing by breathing in and out and take some deep inhales and exhales. It has been noted that people who take a break at around 52 minutes in their work cycle are the most productive people. We became a society of clock-watchers to put in a certain amount of time. Some people are privileged to work by tasks and not the clock.

If you take a long vacation, you are not running away from your responsibilities. Studies show that long breaks from the office reboot your cognitive energy and thus enhance your ability to solve big problems with the mental dexterity required. Take a look at how you can improve your work and productivity by using effective pauses to your day and life.

Eat, Drink and Be Merry...in Your Sleep Time

Health authorities commonly recommend eight 8-ounce glasses of water daily called the 8×8 rule, and it is easy to remember. There are all sorts of theories about the best diets and particular foods that are healthier and plenty of fads. Examine your personal needs and resources and choose wisely. Most people need seven to nine hours of deep sleep to function well and live a healthy life. I have worked with clients via the hypnosis process to help them experience a deeper level of sleep which gave them healthier lives in many other ways. The solution to a busy life is not less sleep. The solution is to have a healthier life style

Read

Work some reading time in to your daily schedule. You may be surprised that once you get on track with this, you can easily read a book a week. Reading gives you new ideas and can change your thoughts and perspectives while deepening your understanding. You can be inspired, entertained and informed to a higher degree.

Plan Your Days and Write Down Your Goals

In writing your goals be sure to get them on paper and be specific. Have deadlines and steps needed to achieve the goal. Be visual. Put up a vision board expressing your goals as a reminder. Revisit your goals and update.

Schedule your days and track them. You might consider setting up or reviewing your week on Sunday or Monday and the next day on the night before. The key is to plan, or your day will take over from other forces and not your own,

Being Present

Being present is not about tasks and data sheets. Quite often it is about our connections, shared humanity and focus. Mastering being in the present can improve social skills, creativity, appreciation, as well as release stress. You can also reduce worry and overthinking and develop a more open and playful spirit.

How can you help yourself to be present? Focus on your breathing. Focus on what is in front of you. Pick up the vibe from people who are present

"The butterfly counts not months but moments and has time enough."

Rabindranath Tagore

Chapter Thirty Two

Who Reads Short Shorts? They're Such Short Shorts

Business Side Up

During my Peace Corps training, I lived with Cate who was a divorced woman living alone. For two months she was my host mother. She had a nice sense of humor, and we maneuvered the language barrier. I was learning Romanian, and she knew little English.

One night, I was asleep and awoke, and I heard male voices and commotion from below my bedroom. The noise was coming from the kitchen which you could only enter by going outside. There was no way to get there from within the rest of the house as it was separate. I believe this had to with convenience during canning and to help control the temperature in the house that could be affected by the use of the kitchen.

I was tired and soon fell back asleep even though the partying continued. My dreams consisted of flashbacks to my high school Latin class, and this was due, I imagine because of my language training The next morning as I walked out of my bedroom to the adjoining room, I was surprised to see several men laying around on the floor sleeping sans clothes. I described the scene to my fellow Peace Corps trainees as that these gentlemen were all "business side up." You go figure that out.

We used that "business side up" expression kind of like a little motto during our tour of duty for other things beyond its original purpose. That evening my host mother explained to me that I did not need to be afraid of these gentlemen who were her relatives. However, their "business side up" presence possibly prompted by a night of drinking and having no idea I was there was a wakeup call just in case I might have been drowsy that day.

On a more serious note, we did have a training video about Siberia. My previous exposure to Siberia had been jokes on late night television about "shipping someone off to Siberia." Sending people to Siberia was something the Soviets did to people that they wanted out of the way. We gained the history and cultural insight to what a reference to Siberia meant to Moldovans. When I was explaining this video in my limited Romanian to my host mother, tears formed in her eyes. Many families suffered the loss and separation of relatives sent to Siberia during the period that Moldova was under the control of the Soviet Union.

Lost in Space

Marta Kristen is a Norwegian-born American actress and is best known for her role as Judy Robinson, one of Professor John and Maureen Robinson's daughters, in the television series *Lost in Space*. Marta was also in charge of lectors at St. Monica Church where I attended. There was an episode of the television show *My Three Sons* titled *Spring Will be a Little Late This Year*. Middle, son Robbie Douglas, played by Don Grady hung out with Marta's character who was a tomboy and skilled in working on cars. Robbie's father encouraged his son to invite the young lady "Pig" on a date. She was all frills and feminine on the date as Peggy and Robbie kissed her at the end of the date. I had a crush on Robbie, and I was not ready for this as a child and I "hated" Pig or Peggy or whatever she was calling herself with her flirtatious ways and screw drivers and wrenches. It was both actors first screen kiss. I told her this story one day in church, and we both got a nice laugh out of it. By the way, years later after watching that particular episode, I became Facebooks friends with both Don and Marta. I tried to get Don to come as a presenter for the Red Carpet Awards. However, he was not able to come. Little did I know he was fighting a battle with cancer at that time. Sadly, Don passed away in June of 2012 on the day I finalized my Peace Corps application.

The Saturday after the Challenger Explosion

Like many people, I was in shock in regard to the explosion of the space shuttle the Challenger on January 28, 1986. I was in disbelief. I had extra interest in astronaut Judy Resnik who was part of the crew. We shared the same hometown of Akron, Ohio and I had attended one of her press conferences

There was to be an exhibition at the California Science Center featuring Judy Resnik coincidentally the Saturday following the Challenger explosion. I had planned to attend, but now my attendance had a deeper meaning. Standing at the exhibit, a woman began talking to me. That is how I met Jeanie Cunningham who then played guitar in Lionel Ritchie's band, and he was very popular at that time

Jeanie had a great admiration for Judy Resnik and even named her recording studio Resnik One as an honor and recorded a song dedicated to Judy. A talented composer and musician Jeanie had a keen interest in space and the astronauts. Later on, in the late 1980s and early 90's she was anonymously responsible for several musical wakeup broadcasts to Space Shuttle astronauts from NASA's mission control earning Jeanie the nickname "The

Most Flown Unknown." I assume that for some reason NASA did not book a rooster. That kind of upset roosters in the world, but I am sure like always Jeanie had some great music.

Jeanie has had a multi-faceted, and inspirational musical career. We were lucky to have her lend her talents to the Red Carpet Awards on a couple of occasions. Our meeting was just one of those accidents in life that bore fruit to a lovely and long friendship.

Germany or Bust

Fellow Peace Corps volunteer Ann Larrow and I had a nice opportunity to travel to Germany for a seminar and training in Dec. of 2014.

The weather was awful. The taxi cabs refused to come to my host mother's house which was as I described it "over the river and through the woods" and with bumpy unpaved roads to boot.

I gave it a shot to try to get other public ground transportation. That was a bit of a hike and on the icy road I fell three times. Seeing stars as I looked up from the pavement after a fall convinced me to return home. In the third fall my phone disappeared into the night and there was no way to locate it. So now the plot thickened that I did not have a phone.

I finally made it to a meeting place and in all the trauma discovered I did not have my passport and had to return to get it. I was pretty sure charm was not going to work with border agents.

Ann and I did make it to the airport and settled in for a long wait. There were few passengers on our flight, and we did finally make it to Germany to join in the seminar. We were the only Americans.

The organizing group was danet: danube networkers for europe. Yes, they used lower case for their organization title. The organization wanted participants from all the countries that bordered Europe. Moldova did actually border the Danube though ever so slightly compared to other countries participating. The event was held in Bad Urach, Germany and the purpose was "Qualification Training aimed at strengthening the civil society and collaboration in the Danube region by capacity building. Countries on the registration list included Servia, Croatia, Slovenia, Germany, Bulgaria, Hungary, the Republic of Moldova (that was us!), Ukraine, Romania, Lithuania, Poland, Albania, and Italy. More than 60 individuals represented about 50 different organizations. The program was interesting and rich in diversity.

We had a harrowing experience getting to the airport to leave for the seminar, but yet a unique cultural experience that led to connections, especially for Ann. It was memorable and eventful, and on my return trip, I had a few hours to see downtown Vienna. It is a beautiful city but even more so when decorated for Christmas.

There are many times in life and not just referencing travel the getting there is tough, but the rewards are memorable and sweet. Bad Urach—well nothing bad about it! Even though the trip got off on a rocky start—not so bad after all.

Save Me A Seat

I had many opportunities in Los Angeles to attend special events. Let me share a few with you. My annual (maybe it happened just once) Magic Night at the Magic Castle in Hollywood. You need to be a member. A female magician friend who performs there graciously worked something out with me, and I would bring a group in. I had a chance to interview some magicians and review their shows as well. Sorry, never got any of the secrets. I was often in awe of things happening on the stage.

Someone contacted me for a women's organization related to the entertainment industry sponsored event and offered free tickets. I was expecting two tickets, but they gave me 50. I had a short time to invite people and did not use all the tickets. I gave it my best shot. It was one of those events that went beyond your expectations as an award show and included dinner.

I went early because I was not sure of some things and wanted to make life as easy as possible for my guests. Perhaps Mickey Rooney had the same idea as we were sitting at adjoining tables and pretty much no one else was around. Lots of people showed up at the last minute. It was beyond what any of us were expecting and considered myself and my guests lucky. Not even sure how my name was on the contact list.

I was invited a few times for events related to the Los Angeles High School for the Performing Arts. Here again, the night was a big surprise. My friend Pam Brealey picked me up, and we made it to downtown LA in record time and got a prime parking space. I was floored that we received seats in the first row close enough to touch Josh Groban, Bob Newhart, Barry Manilow and many other performers and students on hand for this entertainment and awards program. I was thankful for the opportunity and it was a magical night and very exciting.

At a trade show I was attending in Los Angeles for my employer there were some entertainment sessions. Lilly Tomlin was performing in conjunction with the event. I had seen her perform *The Search for Signs of Intelligent Life in the Universe in* my first year living in Los Angeles.

The material that Lilly Tomlin performed was all very fresh to me. One story particularly mesmerized me as to its meaning. I have not been able to find out anything about it.

The story revolves around the comings and goings of life. Off to school, career, marriage and more. The father shares a moment with his son as he goes off for news things in life. The advice is "don't talk about anything spiritual." Then, in turn, the son is now the father, and as his son leaves for the inevitable life changes, he talks to his own son and says "don't' talk about anything spiritual." My friend who I attended the program with had a different opinion that I did. I felt it was about that we don't take the time or put the depth in for life lessons and changes or discuss the spiritual journey. Even in the most important times we get caught up in the color of the wedding gone or the types of appetizers yet miss the spiritual discussion. If anyone is familiar with this piece or has any thoughts, please share them and contact me.

The Facts of Life

My first year in Los Angeles, I met actor/writer Phil Hall. His grandmother was Elizabeth Kerr who played the role of Mindy's grandmother on *Mork and Mindy* starring *Robin Williams* and Pam Dawber. His grandmother was going to be appearing on The Facts of Life television show and he invited me to go to the taping. We had fun and got to go onstage after the taping was complete. I met actress Charlotte Rae.

A short time later, I was invited to a special gala entertainment and awards program that included entertainment performers, sports stars and Olympians. There was a long list of celebrities and a fantastic party afterward with the most elegant tables of food that I have ever seen. I was happy to partake of the delicacies while some celebs posed for pictures and felt a need to refrain from some of the food or they might bust out of their dress.

I did not feel the need to refrain. Interesting that I chatted with Charlotte Ray that night as she remembered me. She was looking for her date. He was probably getting some of that great food.

For years I lived in Toluca Lake very close to Universal Studios. I often enjoyed sitting out on my patio at my condo enjoying the fireworks Universal was shooting off for special events.

I had a long black dress that I kept ready to go in my closet. On occasion, I would get invited to some community dinners and events to be held at Universal to fill out a table. I was close by, and my dress was ready to go with a different jacket, or a new scarf, but always the same dress. I got my money's worth from that and more. You need to keep a dress at the ready because you never know. That is a fact of life.

Several years after the *Facts of Life* taping, I was invited to Elizabeth Kerr's 80th birthday party attended by many friends, relatives of Elizabeth as well as cast and crew from *Mork and Mindy*. I was happy to share in this milestone moment.

A Minor Consideration

I attended some programs of the Entertainment Fellowship a spiritually based group for people involved in entertainment and media established by Robert Hanley also known as Broadway Bob. Robert was a singer/writer/actor. That asked me to get more involved and I helped out on a few things. I had an opportunity to interview Paul Peterson known for playing the character of Jeff on the *Donna Reed Show*.

Paul had been active in helping young performers via an organization he established. *A Minor Consideration* was formed by the efforts of Paul Petersen as a non-profit support and assistance foundation to aid former child stars.

If it had been years before and I had been a teenager I might have been a bit ga-ga. While interviewing Paul over the phone, a minor consideration for me was that I had to go to the bathroom. Well, I worked it out that I gave him a question that would take a while to answer. In the meantime, I multi-tasked and accomplished all of my goals. Paul Peterson's work for young performers deserves a great deal of praise for the help and consideration it has given to transitioning young performers.

Robert Hanley's *Entertainment Fellowship* added a needed spiritual core and I was privileged to be in one of the group's Christmas shows and to lead a discussion group when Robert was ill. Some nice moments that added to my experience.

To A Rose

Kathryn Rose Elick Coffman was a master floral designer in Ohio. While I lived in Los Angeles, Kathy was my go to person for plants and floral arrangements for my mother and other relatives. She went out of her way to make things perfect.

In January of 2005, just a few days after I returned to Los Angeles from Ohio at Christmas time, my father Edmund went to the hospital and then after a few days he was sent to the hospice center and then moved to heaven.

When I first got word of my father going to the hospital and time looking short, I contacted Kathy to find out a polka CD to put with a planter. I had made up some funny titles for songs and emailed this to her. It was not easy for her to find a polka recording. One night, she was at a local store while waiting for her grandson's basketball practice to end. She went through the stack, and no polka CD was there. Rock, rap, country western, oldies, but no polka. She asked the clerk, and the clerk could not be of any help. One more time Kathy looked through the stack and in just a few CDs in the rack there was a polka choice! The angels had to have slipped it in. Kathy bought the CD and placed in with a plant arrangement and sent it to the hospice center and it arrived shortly after my father was admitted.

In April, I began to think I had never received a bill for that planter and CD. It did not appear on any charge card statement. I called Kathy's shop to inquire about this, knowing that she did not want me to deal with this. Oddly the phone just rang with no answer. This seemed odd. I discovered the next day that shortly before my call she had had a stroke and death was imminent. The family was setting up organ donation procedures.

We had always sort of had a joke that neither of us ever called at the right time. She would forget about the time difference from Los Angeles to Ohio and call me at 5 am. I would call at lunchtime in LA which was school pickup time in Ohio. On that day I called just after the family had taken her to the hospital.

When I had been in Ohio in January, I met Kathy for breakfast the day after my father's funeral. She was the florist for the funeral. I brought the funeral program, and we discussed that it had been my father's last Christmas and New Year's. Little did I know as we discussed funerals and life that it had also been her last Christmas and New Year's as well. The thoughts about funerals would soon be very real for her and her large family. But who knew?

There was a garden established at St. Vincent-St. Mary High School in Akron, Ohio near the football field honoring Kathy and a few others. She was a Rose not only in her middle name, not only as a florist but as a person, she was a True Rose in Life.

"For success attitude is equally as important as ability."

Walter Scott

167

Chapter Thirty Three

Take a Giving Vacation -- Out of Africa

In January 2009, I was thinking I would like to go to Ireland that year. I thought the best time for me would be May. I also wanted the trip to be at least partially humanitarian. Two weeks later in my church bulletin, there was a post about a Habitat for Humanity trip to Ireland to help build homes. It was planned for May. Perfect.

Some of the time would be devoted to classes and touring and the opportunity to meet some native Irish people. In addition, we would be swinging hammers as part of the Irish crew that works for Habitat on a regular basis. Right month, right country, humanitarian and tourism combined. How is that for putting your plans out there, knowing that something will find you in a timely manner? No, it does not always work but it does often enough to keep you surprised.

For me, the trip was a nice opportunity to share the experience with others and to work and play with people with a common goal. I learned much about the political situation in Northern Ireland. I am not very handy or mechanical, but I received the necessary instruction to hammer nails and put a roof on a house and perform other duties as well. We had fun with dancing and parties. We sang songs during our workday. Hard to believe but two on our crew had majored in opera. Each day we had a tea break. The Irish work hard and play hard. You can't ask for anything better than that. Since half of my heritage is Irish, I felt the trip helped me get in touch with my roots.

Years ago, I made what I felt was a lofty goal: to travel to all 50 states, visit the inhabited continents and go to 30 countries. At this juncture, just a trip to Australia would make this complete. I went to all 50 states and have visited more than 40 countries. It was comparatively cheap, as I analyze it. This of course was done over quite a few years. I would have never guessed I could do this, but once you have a goal and keep it in mind, you work it out and opportunities sometimes find out about it and come to you. Some travel was work-related, some trips were humanitarian, and with some I just lucked out.

I went to hostels and occasionally camped. A night on the bus or train may have been a sleepover. I found some great travel bargains and cheap flights on my return trip from the Peace Corps to America. That took time and diligence, but it was fun to explore the European bargains for flights.

You may not make all your goals but will have fun trying or adjusting. People who never plan and never set goals get just that — an unplanned life with no clear path and no direction.

As I continue work on this book, I returned from Kenya, in Africa the summer of 2018. While living in Los Angeles I belonged to a fantastic Catholic Church, St. Monica, located just a couple of blocks from the ocean. Annually a group of parishioners visits a sister parish in Kenya. I was supposed to take this missionary trip in 2014 as part of a vacation while serving in the Peace Corps. As time came near for the trip, the Peace Corps would not let me travel to Kenya. They were preparing to pull out of Kenya due to some political and safety concerns. I am so thankful that it worked out that I participated in this trip in 2018.

We had a remarkable journey of spirituality, service, and insight while also enjoying touristy ventures as well. We helped feed women with neurological disorders at a facility run by the Sisters of Charity who are associated with Mother Teresa. We visited an orphanage where the children had HIV and had lost their mothers to the condition, as well. A special touching moment for me was serving lunch to one of the clients at the Sisters of Charity facility. She seemed to have a permanent small tear on her cheek as if she were crying. Others noticed it as well. It gave me extra pause and awareness and added extra thought to the feeding process of these individuals with neurological and physical needs.

We spent many hours sharing and playing with youth groups, children's classes, adult groups, families and more. We visited a hospital and a seminary and interacted with a wide range of age groups.

I think the trip was a better experience for me in 2018 than it would have been in 2014 due to the timing just being a better fit. I was better able to concentrate on the journey because I did not have to think about my Peace Corps service that I would be returning to. On the road of life, travel permits you to put yourself in new situations, be involved in other cultures, and it is a plus to do some good along the way.

Whether you find yourself just Out of Africa or in your own backyard, make your life a reflective one and enjoy the lessons on your personal marathon of life. You may never have a rooster in your bathroom, but be sure to crow a bit as you share your life stories for others.

Story sharing can enhance awareness and allow us to explore the human condition. Stories can improve human relations, performance, ethics, team spirit, understanding, and more. I hope you have enjoyed my stories and learned some lessons or been reminded of things you already know.

Peace and friendship,

Trish Ostroski

"The world is a book and those who do not travel read only one page."

St. Augustine

Final Thoughts

You may never have a rooster in your bathroom and yet it is likely that life has given you some unexpected event, person, or experience that makes you unique and has provided you with stories to share.

There's a Rooster in My Bathroom was intended as a fun title and is based on one of my experiences of sharing a bathroom with a rooster for a few days while serving in the Peace Corps. But before I let you go here are some thoughts about roosters that may apply to you. My research has somewhat surprised me. You may gain something extra to crow about.

Every twelve years the Chinese Zodiac calendar is dedicated to the rooster; 2017 was such a year.

The rooster is known as a time-keeper of the community. When clocks were non-existent, humans relied on roosters to wake them for the start of another day. Tune in to your inner rooster to get your day started. The rooster signifies the dawn of a new day, fidelity and punctuality. The rooster is identified with gallantry, honesty, confidence, candor, and old-fashioned gusto. Those are a lot of good things. I am almost surprised that my rooster did not kick me out of the bathroom.

A rooster plays an important role in its flock. When it finds food, it will call its flock to eat first. In a similar manner you should look out for and look after the people around you; I hope this book has given you some lessons and reminders.

The rooster has made an impact as a religious symbol as well. There's a story in the Bible about how Jesus prophesied about that Peter, one of his apostles, would betray him. Obviously, Peter found it hard to believe that he would condescend to such a level. The cock crowed three times and thus after this event of Peter's denial of Christ, the rooster became a symbol of responsibility, accountability, due care, and loyalty.

So, when you use the expression "a little birdy told me" if that "bird" was a rooster, you might just have something special to crow about no matter the time of day. It is important to note that a rooster serves as an example for us to emulate since it takes care of others first. So, one day, you too might just be lucky enough to have a rooster in your bathroom.

"The will to win, the desire to succeed, the urge to reach your full potential ... these are the keys that will unlock the door to personal excellence."

Confucius

Acknowledgements

I am very grateful to everyone who made this publication possible. Thanks to all who have been along the journey of life.

At Seventeen
Words and Music by Janis Ian
Copyright (c) 1975 Mine Music Limited
Copyright Renewed
All Rights Administered by Sony/ATV Music Publishing LLC, 424 Church Street, Suite 1200, Nashville, TN 37219
International Copyright Secured   All Rights Reserved
Reprinted by Permission of Hal Leonard LLC

Art-Gary Gvtgrafix

Photo credits: Mark Brown, Gary B. Edstrom, Tim Fitzwater, Bruce Ford, Matthew Fried, Matt Jevne, Joan Considine Johnson, Auburn University, NASA.

Other support and assistance: Tom Bird, Denise Cassino, Paige Gold Esq., John Hodgkinson, Idony Lisle, Donna Velasco, Bill Worth, JetLaunch.

About the Author

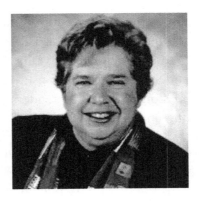

Trish Ostroski has had a varied, interesting life. She served in the United States Peace Corps from 2013-2015 in Moldova in Eastern Europe. It is a former Soviet nation, with approximately three million residents; she had many adventures and powerful experiences while in service there.

Prior to the Peace Corps, Trish was active in the entertainment industry in Hollywood as a playwright, theatrical reviewer, performer, writer, and speaker. While in Los Angeles, she also worked in advertising with video, print, radio, television, and more. Yes, that degree in Mass Media and Communications from the University of Akron eventually paid off.

With more than 500 articles published in newspapers and magazines, she also co-authored a few books, and performed standup comedy at the famous Ice House in Pasadena. She has shared the stage with Joan Van Ark, Lee Meriwether, Lainie Kazan, and Debbie Reynolds.

Trish Ostroski switched gears by training to become a hypnotherapist. Somewhere in the middle, she survived the Northridge Earthquake, lost her car, dealt with her condo that became rubble that fateful day in January of 1994 and lost lots of stuff. In reflection, it was just another journey in life's marathon.

She has served on numerous school, church, community, and professional boards and is currently an Ambassador for the International Cities of Peace in Dayton, Ohio. She writes books that help people understand the world a little more clearly by sharing lessons and stories to enable readers to live their lives with greater meaning and purpose.

She is a certified Jack Canfield Trainer and is available for speaking engagements and training programs. She offers hypnosis sessions for career, health, creativity and sports performance in person or via phone or Skype.

Website: www.wakeupyourlifenow.com
Email: trish@wakeupyourlifenow.com
Phone number: 234-205-1097   330-217-1484

Her book, *There's a Rooster in My Bathroom*, details many wonderful stories and experiences that few others have. Trish currently lives in Ohio near the scenic Cuyahoga Valley National Park.